THIRD EDITION

Subjective Refraction
and **Prescribing Glasses**

The Number One (*or Number Two*) Guide
to Practical Techniques and Principles

THIRD EDITION

Subjective Refraction and Prescribing Glasses

The Number One (*or Number Two*) Guide to Practical Techniques and Principles

RICHARD J. KOLKER, MD
Assistant Professor of Ophthalmology
Johns Hopkins University School of Medicine
Wilmer Eye Institute
Johns Hopkins Hospital
Baltimore, Maryland

ANDREW F. KOLKER, MD
Private Practice
Clinton, Maryland

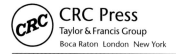

CRC Press
Taylor & Francis Group
Boca Raton London New York

CRC Press is an imprint of the
Taylor & Francis Group, an **informa** business

First Published in 2018 by SLACK Incorporated

Published 2024 by CRC Press
2385 NW Executive Center Drive, Suite 320, Boca Raton FL 33431

and by CRC Press
4 Park Square, Milton Park, Abingdon, Oxon, OX14 4RN

CRC Press is an imprint of Taylor & Francis Group, LLC

Cover Artist: Lori Shields

Dr. Richard J. Kolker and *Dr. Andrew F. Kolker* have no financial or proprietary interest in the materials presented herein.

Original illustrations were produced by the Department of Art as Applied to Medicine, The Johns Hopkins University School of Medicine, Baltimore, Maryland, USA and with a Johns Hopkins University copyright (©JHU).

This book contains information obtained from authentic and highly regarded sources. While all reasonable efforts have been made to publish reliable data and information, neither the author[s] nor the publisher can accept any legal responsibility or liability for any errors or omissions that may be made. The publishers wish to make clear that any views or opinions expressed in this book by individual editors, authors or contributors are personal to them and do not necessarily reflect the views/opinions of the publishers. The information or guidance contained in this book is intended for use by medical, scientific or health-care professionals and is provided strictly as a supplement to the medical or other professional's own judgement, their knowledge of the patient's medical history, relevant manufacturer's instructions and the appropriate best practice guidelines. Because of the rapid advances in medical science, any information or advice on dosages, procedures or diagnoses should be independently verified. The reader is strongly urged to consult the relevant national drug formulary and the drug companies' and device or material manufacturers' printed instructions, and their websites, before administering or utilizing any of the drugs, devices or materials mentioned in this book. This book does not indicate whether a particular treatment is appropriate or suitable for a particular individual. Ultimately it is the sole responsibility of the medical professional to make his or her own professional judgements, so as to advise and treat patients appropriately. The authors and publishers have also attempted to trace the copyright holders of all material reproduced in this publication and apologize to copyright holders if permission to publish in this form has not been obtained. If any copyright material has not been acknowledged please write and let us know so we may rectify in any future reprint.

Library of Congress Cataloging-in-Publication Data

Names: Kolker, Richard J., author. | Kolker, Andrew F., 1981- author.
Title: Subjective refraction and prescribing glasses : the number one (or
  number two) guide to practical techniques and principles / Richard J.
  Kolker, Andrew F. Kolker.
Description: Third edition. | Thorofare : SLACK Incorporated, 2018. |
  Includes index.
Identifiers: LCCN 2018022977 (print) |
ISBN 9781630915599 (pbk.: alk. paper)

Subjects: | MESH: Refraction, Ocular | Refractive Errors--diagnosis |
  Refractive Errors--therapy | Eyeglasses | Prescriptions | Case Reports
Classification: NLM WW 300 | DDC   617.7/55--dc23

LC record available at https://lccn.loc.gov/2018022977

ISBN: 9781630915599 (pbk)
ISBN: 9781003526612 (ebk)

DOI: 10.1201/9781003526612

DEDICATION

Dedicated with love to my wife, Susie, and my children, Andy, David, Jon, and Abby.

Richard J. Kolker, MD

Dedicated, with love and gratitude, to my wife, Grace, and my father, Dr. Richard Kolker.

Andrew F. Kolker, MD

CONTENTS

ACKNOWLEDGMENTS

Our heartfelt thanks and sincere gratitude to:

- David Guyton, MD, for the time, energy, expertise, and attention to detail he gave to this endeavor. Dr. Guyton reviewed the entire manuscript, making helpful corrections to content, wording, and grammar. Without his encouragement, this book would not exist.

- Tony Schiavo, Dani Malady, Allegra Tiver, Michelle Gatt, and Nathan Quinn of SLACK Incorporated. Working with each was a pleasure, and we are especially grateful for their openness to our thoughts and ideas. Their expertise was invaluable in the preparation of this *Third Edition*.

- Laura Ryan, the American Academy of Ophthalmology, for her masterful and caring editing of the original manuscript.

- Scott K. Schultz, MD, for his kind and thoughtful comments and suggestions.

- J. P. Dunn, MD and Michael V. Boland, PhD, for teaching opportunities during resident orientation.

- Cathy Taylor, for arranging resident teaching and for always brightening my day.

- Albert Jun, MD, PhD, for teaching opportunities with medical students.

- Lindsay Beswick, for arranging medical student teaching.

- Mike Hartnett, COT, for suggestions, enthusiasm, and providing teaching opportunities with ophthalmic technicians.

- Joseph Dieter, Johns Hopkins Medical Art Department, for drawing the initial figures that accompany the text.

- Eileen Lesser, for typing the first draft of the manuscript.

- All those from whom I have learned: teachers, colleagues, residents, medical students, ophthalmic technicians, and my patients.

- And special thanks to Bertha Friedberg, Kenneth Greif, Robert Steinberg, Tony Wallace, Paula Massad and Doctors Morton Goldberg, Peter McDonnell, Oliver Schein, Paul Cunningham, Amos Aduroja, Aaron Rabinowitz, Sharon Pusin, Kimberly Williams Bolar, Robert Liss, Steven Pinson, Jack Prince, Eric Singman, Philip Levin, Robert Schreter, and Marshall Levine.

ABOUT THE AUTHORS

Richard J. Kolker, MD is an Assistant Professor of Ophthalmology at the Wilmer Eye Institute of Johns Hopkins Hospital.

Dr. Kolker has taught refraction at the American Academy of Ophthalmology and the Joint Commission of Allied Health Personnel in Ophthalmology Annual Meetings.

His awards include the Wilmer Resident Teaching Award, the Wilmer Medical Student Teaching Award (three-time recipient), the Johns Hopkins School of Nursing Nurse Practitioner Program Best Course of Year Award (two-time recipient), and the University of Maryland School of Nursing Nurse Practitioner Program Best Course of Year Award.

Dr. Kolker's hobbies include teaching refraction, tennis (former Maryland State Champion and member of the University of Pennsylvania tennis team), oldies music, studying religion, singing, theater, and travel. He lives in Baltimore, Maryland with his wife and cocker spaniel. They have four children.

Andrew F. Kolker, MD is a comprehensive ophthalmologist who practices in Clinton, Maryland.

He received his undergraduate degree from University of Pennsylvania, where he graduated *summa cum laude* with a BA in English. He completed his post-baccalaureate pre-medical training at Johns Hopkins University and received his medical degree from Sackler School of Medicine in Tel Aviv, Israel. He completed his internship at Maryland General Hospital and his ophthalmology residency at The George Washington University.

In his free time, Dr. Kolker enjoys creative writing, listening to music, and playing drums and guitar. Tennis is also a passion of his and, as an undergraduate, he was a 4-year varsity tennis letter winner and was co-captain of the team during his senior year.

Following college, Dr. Kolker played tennis professionally, earning a world ranking in singles and doubles. He lives with his wife, Grace, in Washington, DC.

PREFACE

A journey of a thousand miles begins with a single step.
—Lao-tzu, *The Way of Lao-tzu*

It is easy to see that medical and surgical eye care benefit patients in a profound way, at times improving vision in a dramatic fashion. In contrast, it can be easy to overlook that when our patients put on their eyeglasses each morning, vision is improved dramatically. And this improvement is made possible through the process of refraction.

The goal of this manual is to guide the refractionist along the journey of mastering the art of subjective refraction and prescribing glasses. It is an attempt to present this introduction in a clear and accessible manner, with emphasis on the practical.

Subjective refraction can be viewed as simply asking the patient a monotonous series of questions: "Which is more clear, number one or number two?" However, thinking and problem solving are involved continually. When the refractionist understands what is happening optically with each step, the process becomes interesting and can be, at times, quite intellectually challenging. Even after excellently performed retinoscopy or measurement with an autorefractor, subjective refinement is necessary to find the patient's best correction.

Deciding what will be the best glasses prescription for a patient is also an art. The decision is based upon the patient's presenting visual complaint, the result of subjective refraction, and a determination of the reason for the patient's difficulty. This is exactly the same approach with which medical problems are addressed—history, examination, diagnosis, and treatment.

Therefore, it can be seen that subjective refraction and prescribing glasses involve not only measurement, but problem solving. They are the means by which a patient's visual needs are met, as well as determining the best corrected visual acuity. The process, when undertaken with an appreciation of the art and the benefit to the patient, is inherently an enjoyable one.

This book is written to share with the beginning refractionist what I have learned from my teachers, colleagues, students, and patients over 40 years in the practice of ophthalmology. It is my hope that it will be helpful at the beginning of a long and successful career of helping patients with their visual needs.

I'm honored that my son, Dr. Andrew Kolker, has joined me as co-author for this *Third Edition*. It has been an immense pleasure working with him.

Richard J. Kolker, MD

FOREWORD

I believe it was Dr. Frank Newell who said that unless one knows how to obtain best corrected vision, one has no business calling oneself an ophthalmologist. I agree. The process of clinical refraction is the first skill that we teach our residents, and it is the procedure that they are required to repeat more than any other procedure during their training. Best corrected vision, obtained via skillfully performed retinoscopy and subjective refraction, is the primary measure that guides much of our treatment and our surgery. There is no substitute for it.

And yet our patients need more: refractive errors must be corrected. But the practical guidelines and tricks for prescribing glasses, in my experience, are taught neither frequently enough nor well enough. The beginning ophthalmologist is often left to learn these practical points by trial and error, with not enough time, or not enough interest, to engage older colleagues to learn from their wisdom and teaching. Dr. Richard Kolker's text provides simple and elegant exposure to the practical points of subjective refraction and prescribing glasses. He begins with basic terminology and then includes such important topics as the most efficient phrases to use during subjective refraction, the advisability of comparing the new refraction back and forth with the old glasses, the problems patients have adjusting to new glasses, and how to deal with "glasses bounces." An appendix even covers proper use of the lensometer.

The latter half of the text teaches by case examples, an entertaining method of embellishing upon, and adding to, the principles previously presented, in real-world patient situations. The reader is briefly presented with the problem case, has a chance to consider the best solution, and then is taught why the best solution is optimal and why other approaches will likely fail.

The young ophthalmologist will enjoy this text on first reading it and will learn all the more by revisiting it after years of experience. Dr. Kolker has provided our field with a most valuable resource, one that will benefit us and thereby our patients. I heartily recommend it, not only to the beginning ophthalmologist, but to the seasoned ophthalmologist as well.

David L. Guyton, MD
Professor of Ophthalmology
Wilmer Ophthalmological Institute
Baltimore, Maryland

INTRODUCTION

Neither college nor medical school nor anything else prior to entering the field of eye care exposes one to the techniques and principles of refraction. Beginning residents and technicians can, understandably, feel insecure as they begin their journey toward mastery of the art of prescribing glasses. The material in this guide is presented to provide help in taking those first steps.

Chapter 1 discusses the basic optics that enable one to understand the correction of refractive errors and presbyopia. Two important formulas are described, and various types of optical correction are discussed.

Chapter 2 provides the standard method of performing subjective refraction, tips to help with the process, and important considerations before writing the glasses prescription.

Chapter 3 consists of cases in a question-and-answer format. The cases are based on real situations and problems that present to the refractionist, with answers containing techniques and principles important to understand.

An **Appendix** describes how to use the manual lensometer and presents a retinoscopy primer, each in the plus and minus cylinder method.

The emphasis throughout is on the practical. Main points are in **boldface**, and emphasis is given to several by placing them in the upper right corner in large print.

Where plus and minus cylinder techniques differ in Chapter 2 and the Appendix, they are discussed separately. **Black tabs** designate plus cylinder pages and **red tabs** identify minus cylinder pages.

It is our hope that the beginning refractionist will find this guide helpful in understanding, and enjoying, the process of helping patients see more clearly.

Richard J. Kolker, MD
Andrew F. Kolker, MD

CHAPTER 1

Practical Optics

GOAL OF REFRACTION

The ideal refractive state of the eye is **emmetropia** (Figure 1-1). In an **emmetropic** eye, the refractive powers of the cornea and the crystalline lens combine to precisely focus parallel rays of light from a distant object **onto the retina as a single point**. The cornea plays the greater role in achieving this.

Optically, the purpose of refraction is to place a **focal point** onto the retina. Clinically, refraction is how we determine **best corrected visual acuity** as well as the **optimal glasses prescription**; the latter is maximally important to the patient.

The goal of **clinical refraction** is to determine the strength of the corrective lens that will achieve this precise focus when placed in front of the eye. With a well-performed refraction, we are helping our patients see more clearly—**without medicine or surgery**—and they benefit from a correct glasses prescription **all day, every day**!

An eye whose refractive power does not produce this precise focus is **ametropic**, and is described as having a **refractive error**.

◆ Optically, the purpose of refraction is to place a focal point onto the retina.

◆ Clinically, refraction is how we determine best corrected visual acuity as well as the optimal glasses prescription.

Kolker RJ, Kolker AF. *Subjective Refraction and Prescribing Glasses: The Number One (or Number Two) Guide to Practical Techniques and Principles (pp 1-25).*
© 2018 Taylor & Francis Group.

Figure 1-1. Emmetropia. Parallel rays of light from optical infinity focused as a single point on the retina.

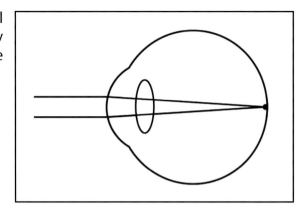

SIX PRINCIPLES OF REFRACTION

1. Refraction is the art of improving vision without medicine or surgery.

2. Refraction and prescribing glasses are best approached as problem solving.

3. The process is more than measurement, and what we measure is not necessarily what we give.

4. History, examination, diagnosis, and treatment decisions are necessary. Just as with medical problems, history plays a large role in determining what will best help the patient.

5. The goal is to give the simplest system that satisfies that individual patient's visual needs.

6. The appropriate prescription is decided upon with each patient. Explain and always show the patient, binocularly, what you are considering prescribing.

Note

After successful eye surgery, a patient with residual refractive error is able to achieve the full benefit of the surgery only when fitted with the proper glasses.

SNELLEN VISUAL ACUITY

What Does 20/20 Vision Mean?

The correction of refractive error is the focusing of parallel rays of light onto the retina. Light rays from optical infinity enter the eye in a parallel fashion, and those from twenty feet are essentially parallel. It is for this reason the visual acuity chart is placed 20 feet from the patient.

Identifying letters on the **Snellen chart** is the classic, and still the most common, way visual acuity is measured. The **ETDRS acuity chart** has also been in use since the commencement of the Early Treatment Diabetic Retinopathy Study in 1979.

The Snellen (or other) visual acuity chart is placed at 20 feet either literally or by way of mirrors. Alternatively, the size of the letters on the chart can be adjusted to achieve essentially the same effect.

The 20/20 designation is based on what the "normal" individual is able to see. A person with normal vision is able to read letters of a given size at 20 feet. **Visual acuity of 20/20 means that the individual can read at 20 feet what the normal person can read at 20 feet**.

The metric equivalent of 20/20 in meters is 6/6.

What Does 20/80 Vision Indicate?

If someone has 20/80 vision, that means the individual has to be 20 feet away to see clearly what the normal person can see from a distance of 80 feet.

Can Vision Be Better Than 20/20?

Yes, some individuals have better than 20/20 visual acuity. If, for example, one has 20/15 acuity, that individual can read from 20 feet away what the normal person could only read at 15 feet.

Is Pinhole Acuity the Same as Best Corrected Visual Acuity?

No, it is not. It is not unusual for refraction to yield better acuity than the pinhole.

SPHERICAL REFRACTIVE ERRORS

There are two types of spherical refractive errors: myopia and hyperopia.

In **myopia**, parallel rays of light from optical infinity, bent by the cornea and the crystalline lens, come to a **focal point in front of the retina**. The eye is "**too long**" relative to its inherent plus power. The patient is described as being **myopic** or **nearsighted**. This is corrected with a biconcave lens—a **minus (red) lens**—which diverges the rays of light so that the focal point moves posteriorly and is focused on the retina (Figure 1-2).

In **hyperopia**, parallel rays of light from optical infinity, bent by the cornea and the crystalline lens, come to a **focal point behind the retina**. The eye is "**too short**" relative to its inherent plus power. The patient is described as being **hyperopic** or **farsighted**. This is corrected with a biconvex lens—a **plus (black) lens**—which converges the rays of light so that the focal point moves anteriorly and is focused on the retina (Figure 1-3).

Myopia and **hyperopia** are corrected by a spherical lens, or **sphere**, of a specific power.

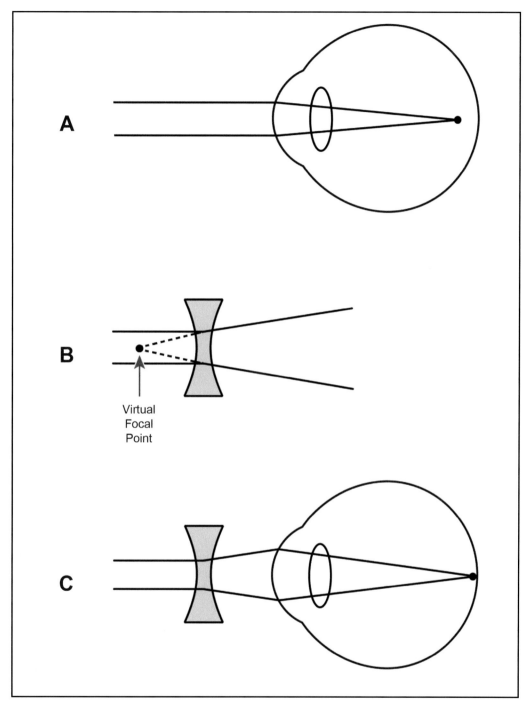

Figure 1-2. Myopia.

A. Parallel rays of light from optical infinity focused as a single point in front of the retina. The eye is "too long."

B. A biconcave (minus) lens diverges rays of light.

C. A minus lens corrects myopia.

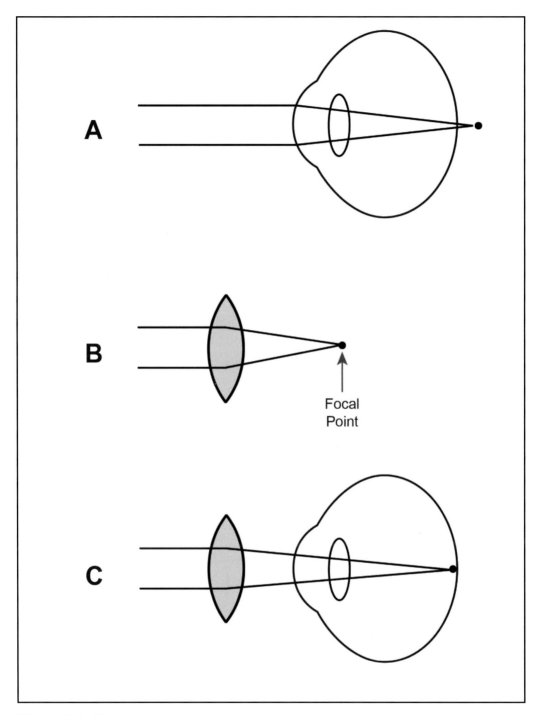

Figure 1-3. Hyperonia.

   A. Parallel rays of light from optical infinity focused as a single point behind the retina. The eye is "too short."

   B. A biconvex (plus) lens converges rays of light.

   C. A plus lens corrects hyperonia.

Fallacy Alert

There is an interesting fallacy in the seemingly straightforward term **farsighted**. When not wearing corrective glasses, a moderately near-sighted person has blurred vision at distance but can see clearly at near; thus, being called **nearsighted**. The term **nearsighted** works: one can see clearly at near, but not at far.

One might then logically conclude that, for a farsighted person, the opposite would be the case—the individual would have blurred vision at near but be able to see clearly at distance. However, this is not so. A moderately farsighted person has blurred vision at distance! Thus, the term **farsighted** is a fallacy because the individual cannot see clearly at far without correction.

The reason this seemingly simple terminology breaks down is that the nearsighted/farsighted designations do not properly describe what is happening with these refractive errors. A camera analogy demonstrates what is occurring in myopia and hyperopia. If a camera is in focus at distance, the image becomes equally blurred if the focusing lens is turned to the right or the left; that is, if the image is defocused anteriorly or posteriorly. **Similarly for the eye, a distant image will be blurred if the focal point is in front of (myopia) or behind (hyperopia) the retina.**

So, should the terms **nearsighted** and **farsighted** be replaced, respectively, with "like a camera whose image is blurred because it is displaced too far anteriorly" and "like a camera whose image is blurred because it is displaced too far posteriorly"? Probably not!

ASTIGMATISM

Astigmatism is a Greek term meaning "**without a point**." Parallel rays of light passing through an astigmatic surface do not come together as a focal point. An eye's astigmatism is mostly due to the **curvature of the cornea**, although the crystalline lens can also contribute. An easy way to understand astigmatism is to consider the difference between a **basketball** and an **American football**. We know that they have different shapes, but we usually do not stop to think about exactly how they are different (Figure 1-4).

A **basketball** has one curvature. Wherever you look, the curvature is the same. A single curvature equates to an optical system that is **spherical**.

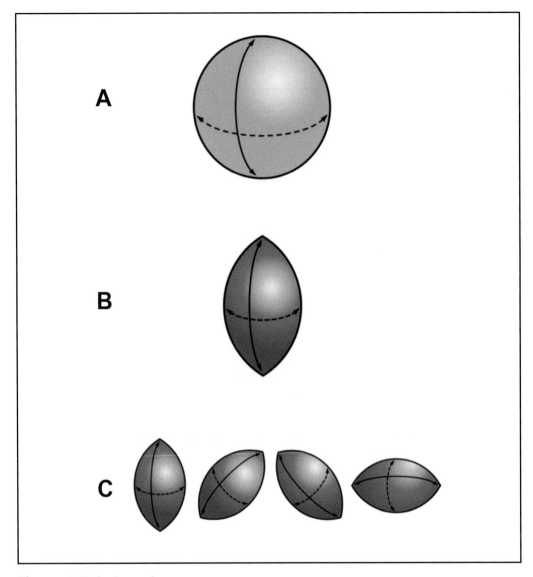

Figure 1-4. Astigmatism.

    A. A "basketball" cornea has no astigmatism. The curvature of the solid line and the broken line are the same.

    B. A "football" cornea has astigmatism. The curvature of the solid line (more gradual) and the broken line (more steep) are not the same.

    C. The angle of the football determines its axis.

An American **football** looks different. This is because it has two curvatures. If we put the football on a table and hold it so that its tip is pointing upward, we can see that it has a gradual curve from top to bottom and a steeper curve from side to side. Two different curvatures equate to an optical system that is **astigmatic**.

- A "basketball" cornea has no astigmatism.
- A "football" cornea has astigmatism.

Thus, a basketball-shaped cornea has no astigmatism, in contrast to a football-shaped cornea, which is astigmatic.

Astigmatism is corrected by a **cylinder** of a specific **power** and orientation. The orientation is called its **axis**. There are two ways the power and axis of the cylinder can be determined: the **plus cylinder method** and the **minus cylinder method**. Just as a given length can be expressed in inches or centimeters, a prescription for glasses can be measured and recorded with plus or minus cylinder power. A plus cylinder prescription can be converted to a minus cylinder prescription, and vice versa (see *Plus-Minus Cylinder Conversion* on page 24).

Either system of notation can be used for an eyeglass prescription. Minus cylinder is used for contact lens prescriptions and for refractive surgery. Plus cylinder is used in the calculations for toric (astigmatism-correcting) intraocular lenses.

Where they differ, the plus and minus cylinder methods are **discussed separately**. The principles of refraction apply equally to both.

Note

In contact lens and intraocular lens terminology, the term **toric** is used to describe a lens correcting for astigmatism.

Axis is another aspect of astigmatism that must also be taken into account. We have described the two curvatures of the football while it is held with the tip pointing upward, but a football can also be held in a variety of tilted positions to the left or right. It can even lie on a table in a horizontal position. The orientation of the football is its axis, which can range from 0 to 180 degrees from the horizontal. An astigmatic cornea is described in the same manner.

An astigmatic cornea that has not been altered by corneal disease will have two curvatures 90 degrees apart; this is termed **regular astigmatism**. Regular astigmatism can be corrected with a cylinder in the glasses prescription. If the shape of a cornea has been altered by corneal disease, it will have more than two curvatures; this is termed **irregular astigmatism**. Irregular astigmatism cannot be fully corrected with a cylinder and, therefore, a rigid contact lens is often used to allow the tear film to fill in the irregularities of the surface.

When parallel rays of light from an object pass through a spherical refracting surface, a single point of focus is the result. However, when parallel light rays pass through a **spherocylindrical system**, a single point of focus is not achieved.

The result is a unique appearing shape, which can be visualized as two ice cream cones joined at their tips, with one cone squashed horizontally and the other vertically. This configuration was first described by J.F.C. Sturm in 1838 and is called the **conoid of Sturm** (Figure 1-5A).

- ◆ When parallel rays of light from an object pass through a spherical refracting surface, a single point of focus is the result.

- ◆ However, when parallel light rays pass through a spherocylindrical system, a single point of focus is not achieved.

If one cuts cross-sections sequentially through the conoid, the result is a series of elliptical images, two focal lines, and a central circle (Figure 1-5B).

The most important parts of the conoid of Sturm are the two focal lines and the circle, the latter always located dioptrically halfway between the two lines. A vertical curvature will produce a horizontal focal line, and a horizontal curvature produces a vertical focal line.

If, to simplify the conoid of Sturm, one ignores the ellipses and looks simply at the two focal lines with the circle in the center, this is called the **interval of Sturm** (Figure 1-5C).

If, further simplifying the conoid of Sturm, one eliminates the ellipses and the two focal lines, only the circle remains. The circle is called the **circle of least confusion** (Figure 1-5D).

Thus, the circle of least confusion can be used to represent the conoid of Sturm, the result of light rays passing through a spherocylindrical surface. The circle of least confusion is also referred to as the **blur circle**. The blur circle is produced by an astigmatic refracting system, in contrast to a point of focus produced by a spherical system. It is always, dioptrically, midway between the two focal lines. The closer the focal lines are to each other, the smaller the blur circle. **The blur circle is the clearest image when astigmatism is not fully corrected.**

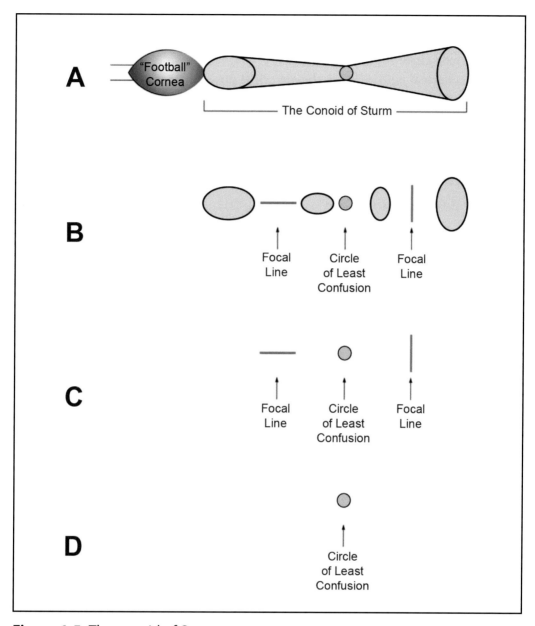

Figure 1-5. The conoid of Sturm.

A. The conoid of Sturm.

B. Cross sections through the conoid of Sturm.

C. A simplification: the interval of Sturm. It is the distance between the two focal lines.

D. Further simplification: the circle of least confusion. It is always dioptrically midway between the two focal lines. It is also referred to as the *blur circle*. When on the retina, it represents the spherical equivalent.

During the process of refraction, the conoid of Sturm and, therefore, the blur circle can be moved anteriorly and posteriorly, just as a focal point's position can be changed. When the blur circle is positioned on the retina, it represents the **spherical equivalent**. **The spherical equivalent is the spherical power that places the circle of least confusion (the blur circle) onto the retina.**

Note

A cylinder's power (its meridian) is 90 degrees from its axis.

A cylinder correcting lens moves the focal line parallel to its axis.

Some beginning optics students jokingly call the center of the conoid of Sturm "the circle of most confusion." It need not be!

Types of Astigmatism

The three types of astigmatism are **simple**, **compound**, and **mixed**. Figure 1-6 contains a definition and diagram of each type.

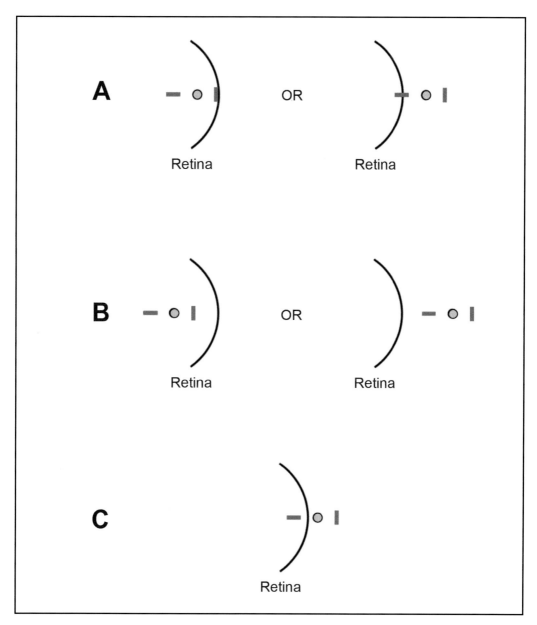

Figure 1-6. Types of astigmatism, demonstrated by the interval of Sturm.

  A. Simple astigmatism: One meridian is emmetropic, the other is either myopic or hyperopic.

  B. Compound astigmatism: Both meridians are myopic or hyperopic.

  C. Mixed astigmatism: One meridian is myopic, the other is hyperopic.

With-the-Rule, Against-the-Rule, and Oblique Astigmatism

▶ **With-the-rule astigmatism**: Corrected with **plus cylinder axis at 90 degrees** OR **minus cylinder axis at 180 degrees**. (More common in a younger patient.)

▶ **Against-the-rule astigmatism**: Corrected with **plus axis at 180 degrees** OR **minus cylinder axis at 90 degrees**. (More common in an older patient.)

▶ **Oblique astigmatism**: Axes other than 90 or 180 degrees; often symmetrical. **Note: When symmetrical, cylinder axes add to 180 degrees.**

Note

Bilateral non-oblique axes also add to **180 degrees**:

Both axes at **90 degrees** equals 180 (90 + 90 = 180).

Both axes at **180 degrees** equals 180 because 180 is also 0 (180 + 0 = 180)!

PRESBYOPIA

The term **presbyopia** comes from the Greek *presbyteros*, which means "old-age vision." It is probably best to refrain from mentioning this derivation to patients!

To understand presbyopia, it is helpful to begin with an analogy to a camera (useful for many aspects of the functioning of the eye). When a camera is in focus for an object in the distance and subsequently needs to take a picture of something up close, a change in focus must occur.

In their resting state, after the correction of any refractive error, our eyes are like a camera set for distance. To view nearer objects clearly, some **focusing** is necessary. The nearer the object, the more focusing is required.

The focusing performed by our eyes for near viewing is called **accommodation**. Accommodation is achieved by an increase in the plus power of our natural crystalline lens. When we look in the distance, the ciliary muscle is relaxed and the taut zonular fibers pull on the crystalline lens. Near viewing is accomplished by circumferential contracture of the ciliary muscle, like a sphincter or purse-string, which loosens the pull of the zonular fibers. This results in the crystalline lens reverting to its more convex shape, thus increasing its plus power.

Presbyopia is the **age-related decrease in accommodative ability** that occurs inevitably in everyone, **whether one is nearsighted, farsighted, or emmetropic**. In childhood, we have a large amount of accommodative ability, but this gradually decreases over our lifetime. By age 45 years, help for seeing clearly at near is usually needed in the form of reading glasses for emmetropes or the addition of a **bifocal or progressive addition lens (PAL)** for those wearing a distance correction.

Presbyopia is treated with **plus power** to make up for the decreasing ability of the natural crystalline lens to become more convex. Initially, when some accommodation remains, the plus corrective lenses are supplementing that residual ability. Eventually, when all useful accommodation is lost, the correction replaces it completely. The added plus power is referred to as the **Reading Addition** or more commonly as the **Add**. The Add is an addition to the lower portion of the distance correction, and its efficacy depends on a **correct distance prescription**. Another way to understand presbyopia is with an extension of the previously mentioned camera analogy. When we are young, our "camera" can focus very rapidly, instantaneously, from distance to near. However, let's say we take our camera to the beach every summer and it gets more and more sand in it each time. Over the years, as the sand accumulates in the camera, it will lose the ability to make those last few turns for focusing up close.

For our patients, when an insufficient amount of accommodation remains for reading at near, they often complain that their "**arms aren't long enough**." They have to push their reading material farther away to see clearly because their loss of accommodative ability (sand in the camera) does not allow them to focus at their normal reading distance (the camera cannot make those last few turns). Reading farther away requires less accommodation.

Fallacy Alert

It is sometimes stated, "**One gets more farsighted as one gets older.**" This is incorrect and results from a misunderstanding of presbyopia. At the onset of presbyopia, one is indeed able to see reading material more clearly by pushing it farther away to a position where less accommodation is needed. However, this is not the same as becoming more farsighted, which is a description of refractive error at distance.

FOUR POINTS ABOUT
CORRECTING PRESBYOPIA WITH AN ADD

The Add is an addition to the lower portion of the distance correction, and its efficacy depends upon a correct distance prescription.

1. The following **rule of thumb** for Add strength is often helpful:

   - **At age 45 years**, the typical Add that is needed is **+1.50 diopters**.

   - **At age 50 years**, the typical Add that is needed is **+2.00 diopters**.

   - **At age 55 years**, the typical Add that is needed is **+2.50 diopters**.

Note

If an appropriate age-related Add is given, but the distance prescription is incorrect, the reading portion of the lens will not be correct.

Although we retain some accommodative ability into our early seventies, the maximal strength Add, typically **+2.50 diopters**, is usually needed by our mid-50s.

At any age, if **cataract surgery** has been performed with a monofocal intraocular lens implant that rendered the eye **emmetropic**, an Add of **+2.50 diopters** is typically given.

For practical purposes, when determining the proper Add to prescribe, have patients hold the near card at their **usual reading distance** rather than at 14 inches as described on the Rosenbaum Pocket Vision Screener. The Rosenbaum card states the card is held at 14 inches from the eye because it is at that position the distance equivalent and Jeager values correspond. However, some individuals prefer to read closer than 14 inches, and others farther. The determination of the proper Add strength should be made at each individual patient's preferred reading distance.

Note

Make sure that when patients are asked to hold the reading card at their preferred reading distance, it is their ideal reading distance and not the distance at which they now "prefer" because of presbyopia.

2. When testing to find which Add to prescribe, it is important to ensure that the lens strength the patient prefers is making the figures on the near card **clearer rather than larger**. This distinction is necessary because if the patient is comparing two choices that give equal clarity, the patient may respond that the choice producing the larger figures is "better." However, the goal of a presbyopic correction is to supplement or replace the accommodative ability that has been lost over time. Before the patient became presbyopic, the patient's accommodative ability brought the reading material into focus but did not magnify it. The purpose of a presbyopic Add is to do the same. Magnification is an indication that the Add is overly strong and will produce a **reading range that is closer and narrower than necessary**. (See *Reading Glasses* on page 19 for a discussion of range of clarity.)

Fallacy Alert

Although it is common for over-the-counter reading glasses to be referred to as **magnifiers**, they should really be called **focusers**. Prior to the onset of presbyopia, the patient's accommodative ability was used to focus, not magnify.

3. When prescribing an Add, testing the **range** in which the vision remains clear can be very helpful. The purpose is to make sure that the Add not only provides clear vision at the patient's ideal reading position, but also nearer and farther than that position.

The reading range is tested by having a patient hold the near card at the preferred reading distance, and then asking that the card be brought **progressively closer, stopping when the figures blur**. The position at which that occurs is the near point of the range. Next, **the card is pushed away** until blurring occurs, that being the far point of the range. An ideal reading range has the preferred reading distance **midway** between these two points.

If reading glasses are going to be used both for close reading and for reading on the computer, it is important to check the range of clarity. Ideally, the range should include the close reading position as well as the computer monitor distance. If it does not, the patient can use separate reading and computer glasses, the latter having less plus power.

Note

Increasing the plus power of an Add results in a closer and narrower reading range. Interestingly, an Add that is **too strong** can produce more difficulty for the patient than an Add that is too weak. Patients are often more distressed about having to hold their reading material too close than they are about having to push it farther away.

4. **Stronger Adds of +3.00, +3.50, or higher** can be given for individuals who prefer an unusually close reading distance or given as a low vision aid with the intention of producing magnification.

- ◆ The stronger the reading glasses, the closer and more narrow the range.
- ◆ The less strong the reading glasses, the less close and the wider the range.

BIFOCALS

The bifocal was invented by **Benjamin Franklin** in the eighteenth century. At that time, when someone wearing glasses became presbyopic, a separate pair of reading glasses was prescribed. When Ben Franklin found himself in that situation, he felt it was inefficient to have to change glasses when alternating his vision from distance to near and vice versa.

Franklin realized that when viewing at distance through his distance glasses, he was using the top portion of the lenses, and when reading at near with the reading glasses, he was using the bottom portion of the lenses. (As is the case with many brilliant observations, they seem quite obvious once made.) Therefore, he decided to cut each distance and reading lens in half and glue them to each other, with the distance lens at the top and the reading lens at the bottom. Thus, he had **two pairs of glasses in one**—and the bifocal was invented!

The top part of a bifocal lens corrects the patient's distance refractive error, and the bottom part of the lens contains that distance correction **combined with additional plus power** for focusing at near. Thus, the lower section in a bifocal is dependent upon and is an **addition to the distance prescription**. The additional plus power is referred to as the **Add**, and its strength is determined by the amount of focusing power needing supplementation by the patient.

Example: For a distance prescription -4.50 +0.75 × 10°, and the need for a +2.50 Add:

- The bifocal prescription would be written as -4.50 +0.75 × 10° (+2.50).
- When the patient is looking at near, the power that the patient is reading with is determined by the **algebraic sum** of the sphere and the Add: -2.00 +0.75 × 10°.

The bifocal segment can be made in several configurations:

- **Flat-top or "standard" bifocal**: The top of the bifocal is a flat line and the segment occupies a portion of the lower part of the lens. Most bifocals "with a line" are of this type.
- **Round or half-moon crescent**: The segment is circular and is often cut off at the bottom of the lens resulting in a half moon shape.
- **Executive**: The line and bifocal segment extend across the entire lower lens.
- **Blended**: No easily visible separation line, but not a PAL.

Note

When using the bifocal segment, the patient is looking through a combination of the distance prescription and the Add. **Therefore, the bifocal segment is dependent upon a distance prescription that is correct.**

READING GLASSES

At times, it is appropriate, based on the patient's needs or preference, to prescribe a separate pair of reading glasses. The reading glasses prescription is determined by **algebraically adding the distance prescription sphere and the reading Add**, leaving any astigmatic correction unchanged.

Example: For the bifocal prescription -4.50 +0.75 × 10° (+2.50):

- The distance prescription is -4.50 +0.75 × 10°.
- The reading glasses prescription is -2.00 +0.75 × 10°.

Note

This is, and should be, the same power the patient is looking through when using the bifocal segment.

Misnomer Alert

A patient will sometimes be surprised to find, "I now need my reading glasses when I'm eating!" The term **reading glasses** is, in a sense, a misnomer. Reading glasses are really "**near glasses.**" They are making up for the focusing that we are no longer able to do for any **near task, not just reading**.

TRIFOCALS

Trifocals are an extension of Ben Franklin's concept for the bifocal, incorporating a third lens for correction of the **intermediate distance**. The standard bifocal, with a line separating the distance and the near portions of the lens, allows for clear vision both at distance and at near. Objects in the intermediate distance (the area beyond the normal reading distance and less than 20 feet away) are not seen clearly through either the top or bottom of the bifocal. (Thus, to view something at the intermediate distance when using a standard bifocal, one must either come closer and use the bifocal segment, or back away and use the distance portion of the lens.) The trifocal adds a **third lens** between the distance and near portions of the standard bifocal to correct for the intermediate distance. There are three lenses combined into one, with two lines separating the three segments.

The power written for the trifocal is typically **one-half the strength of the bifocal Add**, although other strengths can be designated.

Example: For the bifocal prescription -4.50 +0.75 × 10° (+2.50):

- One-half the bifocal Add is +1.25.
- The trifocal prescription would be -4.50 +0.75 × 10° (+1.25) (+2.50).

Note

Since the advent of the PAL, trifocals are prescribed much less frequently as the solution to viewing the intermediate distance.

PROGRESSIVE ADDITION LENSES

The standard bifocal works well for far and close viewing, but it does not provide for clear vision in the intermediate area between distance and near. The trifocal has a third lens that allows for clarity at the intermediate distance, but there are still gaps—one between the distance and intermediate area, and another between intermediate and near. The **progressive addition lens (PAL)** is an extension of the bifocal and trifocal concepts. It can be thought of as a **graduated multifocal. The distance correction is at the top of the lens, and plus power increases progressively in the lower portion of the lens until the prescribed Add power is reached.** Thus, one can focus clearly, progressively, from distance to near; there are no gaps.

Note

The PAL is sometimes called a **no-line bifocal**, and some patients refer to it incorrectly as a **trifocal**.

Most patients consider the "no line" a cosmetic benefit.

When the PAL is working properly, distance vision is corrected with the normal straight-ahead head position, near is corrected with the normal eyes-down reading position, and the intermediate distance is corrected with varying amounts of chin-up positioning depending on how far away an object is. The closer the object is in the intermediate distance, the more elevated the chin needs to be. When patients are using the PAL successfully, their functioning should be similar to how it was before they became presbyopic. They are able to **see clearly at distance and near, as well as all points in between**, seamlessly.

Note

With a **desktop computer**, the monitor screen is often in the intermediate distance, and it is brought into clear focus with a **slight chin-up position**.

The PAL does have a special consideration resulting from the way the graduation is achieved in the grinding of the lens; there is an **inherent blur at the sides**. One must be looking straight ahead for clear viewing. However, as progressive lenses manufacturing has improved, the clear central channel and reading areas have been widened. This has made adjustment to, and functioning with, the PAL much easier. The introduction of the **free-form progressive lens** has been a significant advance in this regard.

Note

Many individuals were taught in school to move their eyes across the line of print when reading. With the PAL, one may need to move one's head when reading in order to keep looking through the central part of the lens. It is surprising how easily most people are able to make this change—and especially surprising after all of those years of moving only their eyes! Most individuals are able to adjust to the progressive lens right away, although for some, it can take up to 2 weeks. It is quite helpful to explain this to the patient when prescribing the first PAL.

COMPUTER GLASSES

With both a trifocal and a PAL, it is necessary to adopt a slight chin-up position to view a desktop computer screen because it is typically located at the intermediate distance. Some individuals cannot or prefer not to work in that position; in these situations, separate computer glasses may be given.

The top portion of computer glasses corrects for the intermediate distance, not for 20 feet and beyond as in a normal bifocal, trifocal, or PAL. The bottom portion of computer glasses can have a correction for near, given either as a bifocal segment or a PAL, the latter having the advantage of allowing clear vision progressively from the intermediate distance to near. A **bifocal or PAL** is often preferable to a single vision intermediate lens because without the correction for near, there can be difficulty reading something printed from the computer or other reading material.

The computer glasses prescription is calculated by **splitting the patient's normal Add in half**. One-half of the Add is incorporated into the top part of the lens, leaving the remaining half of the Add at the bottom part of the lens. This will result in an **odd-looking Add power** when the prescription is written.

The Calculation

To have the intermediate distance correction at the top of the lens, the Add is divided in half. **One-half of the strength of the full Add is added to the distance sphere algebraically**; this will determine the top portion of the computer glasses. **The remaining half of the strength of the full Add is written as the Add for the computer glasses.** This will result in the full reading power being present in the bottom portion of the computer glasses.

> ### *Note*
> One way to check that the computer glasses prescription has been calculated correctly is by making certain the total reading power is correct.

Example: If the bifocal prescription is -4.50 +0.75 × 10° (+2.50):

- The power for the top half of the computer glasses is obtained by adding one-half of the bifocal strength, +1.25, to the distance prescription: -3.25 +0.75 × 10°.

- The remainder of the bifocal strength, +1.25, becomes the Add for the computer glasses, resulting in a prescription of: -3.25 +0.75 × 10° (+1.25).

- It is only the top portion of the computer glasses that differs in total power from the patient's regular bifocal. The reading portion in the computer glasses (the **odd-looking Add** added algebraically to the sphere) has the same power as the regular bifocal: -2.00 +0.75 × 10°.

TWO FORMULAS: SPHERICAL EQUIVALENT AND PLUS-MINUS CYLINDER CONVERSION

For everyday clinical practice, it is necessary to know the following two formulas: spherical equivalent and plus-minus cylinder conversion.

Spherical Equivalent of an Astigmatic Prescription

An astigmatic eye requires a prescription with spherical power and cylinder power at a specified axis; this combination results in a focal point positioned on the retina. The cylinder axis and power are correcting the astigmatic part of the refractive error.

If an astigmatic eye were to be corrected with a spherical lens alone, the result would be a blur circle (a **circle of least confusion**). The spherical lens power that places the circle of least confusion on the retina is called the **spherical equivalent**.

The rule for finding the spherical equivalent: Add one-half of the cylinder power to the sphere algebraically (that is, keeping in mind the plus and minus signs).

Example 1: What is the spherical equivalent of -6.00 +2.00 × 90°?

- **Applying the rule**: One-half of the cylinder power is +1.00; +1.00 added algebraically to -6.00 = -5.00.

- **Answer**: -5.00.

When writing a glasses prescription, the spherical equivalent calculation is used if one decides to give less cylinder power than was measured. If it was decided to reduce the cylinder power in this example by one-half of a diopter, the resulting prescription would be: -5.75 +1.50 × 90°. This calculation can and should be checked by making sure the original and the modified prescriptions have the **same spherical equivalent (-5.00)**.

Example 2: What is the spherical equivalent for +4.00 -0.50 x 180°?

- **Applying the rule**: One-half of the cylinder power is -0.25; -0.25 added algebraically to +4.00 = +3.75.

- **Answer**: +3.75.

Plus-Minus Cylinder Conversion

It is necessary to know how to convert a glasses prescription from plus cylinder to minus cylinder, and vice versa.

There are three steps:

1. **Add the cylinder power to the sphere algebraically, taking into account the plus and minus signs.**

2. **Change the sign of the cylinder from plus to minus, or from minus to plus.**

3. **Change the axis by 90 degrees (i.e., add or subtract 90 degrees).**

Example 1: -4.00 -2.00 × 65°.

- In plus cylinder form, it equals -6.00 +2.00 × 155°.

Example 2: +3.50 -1.50 × 115°.

- In plus cylinder form, it equals +2.00 +1.50 × 25°.

Example 3: -4.25 +1.25 × 90°.

- In minus cylinder form, it equals: -3.00 -1.25 × 180°.

Note

It is good to check the correctness of a conversion by reconverting to the original cylinder sign.

PINHOLE

Visual acuity can be measured with the patient looking through a pinhole aperture, typically 1.2 mm in diameter. The pinhole is placed directly in front of the patient's eyeglass lens (or eye if the patient is not wearing glasses). **If visual acuity improves with the pinhole, this indicates there may be uncorrected refractive error.** The pinhole may also improve vision if there is ocular surface disease, irregular astigmatism, cataract, or other media or retinal abnormalities. **If visual acuity does not improve with the pinhole, refraction may result in improvement.**

Historically, the pinhole was used to assess acuity when an individual presented to the emergency department with broken or lost glasses. In modern times, pinhole acuity is sometimes used as a surrogate for best vision, but it does not always indicate the best acuity the patient may have. **Best corrected visual acuity is determined by refraction.**

CHAPTER 2

Subjective Refraction and Lens Prescription

THE PHOROPTER

Subjective refraction begins with the result from **retinoscopy**, **autorefraction**, or the patient's **current glasses**. When no prior information is available, subjective refraction can begin **de novo**.

When starting de novo ("from the beginning") two methods can be used to determine if cylinder is present. (See *Sixteen Tips for Accurate Subjective Refraction Results, Tip 9* on page 64.)

The patient's refinement of the starting point is necessary to arrive at the best correction for the refractive error, even when retinoscopy is performed expertly or a modern autorefractor is used.

The starting prescription is dialed into the refractor, usually referred to as a **phoropter** or by the identical sounding trade name, Phoroptor (Reichert Technologies). Alternatively, loose lenses or lenses put in a trial frame can be used when a phoropter is unavailable or for a patient unable to cooperate. The phoropter is a collection of these lenses, with excellent design to provide greater ease and convenience for the refractionist (Figure 2-1).

Kolker RJ, Kolker AF. *Subjective Refraction and Prescribing Glasses: The Number One (or Number Two) Guide to Practical Techniques and Principles (pp 27-74).*
© 2018 Taylor & Francis Group.

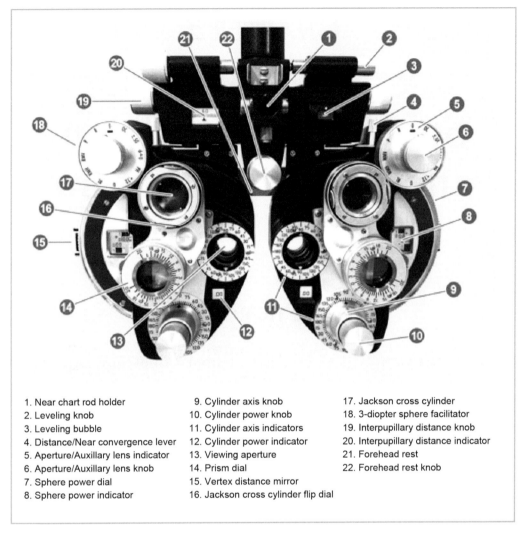

Figure 2-1. Phoropter.

1. Near chart rod holder
2. Leveling knob
3. Leveling bubble
4. Distance/Near convergence lever
5. Aperture/Auxillary lens indicator
6. Aperture/Auxillary lens knob
7. Sphere power dial
8. Sphere power indicator
9. Cylinder axis knob
10. Cylinder power knob
11. Cylinder axis indicators
12. Cylinder power indicator
13. Viewing aperture
14. Prism dial
15. Vertex distance mirror
16. Jackson cross cylinder flip dial
17. Jackson cross cylinder
18. 3-diopter sphere facilitator
19. Interpupillary distance knob
20. Interpupillary distance indicator
21. Forehead rest
22. Forehead rest knob

Features of the Phoropter

▶ **Sphere power dial**: Whether one is working in the plus or minus range, pulling down is adding plus power and pushing up is adding minus power.

► **Jackson cross cylinder** (JCC): When lowered into position, it clicks into place. Likewise, when its dots are in proper position (straddling or on axis), they click into place. When changing from the straddling position to the on axis position, turn the JCC clockwise. There are two sets of corresponding

The arrows on the small and large cylinder axis indicators correspond and move together.

dots and arrows; choose one set to work with (the set more easily seen). The JCC has two flip dials; pick the one most comfortable to use, and always turn it in the same direction, even when repeating choices.

► **Cylinder axis indicators** (one large, one small): The degrees are marked from 0 to 180, matching above and below the horizontal. The large and small axis indicators correspond to each other, with the larger marked in 5-degree increments and the smaller in 15-degree increments. When the JCC is clicked into position, it is in front of the smaller axis indicator.

► **Cylinder axis knob**: It has two arrows 180 degrees apart, each indicating the axis on the larger cylinder axis indicator. This knob turns three things: its two arrows, the two arrows of the smaller cylinder axis indicator, and the JCC. All three are synchronized.

Note

Hand-held JCCs are also available. They come in .25-diopter steps up to 1 diopter, both in plus and minus cylinder.

The **JCC** has been known to instill dread in some beginning refractionists. Just the opposite should be the case. This brilliant two-in-one little lens will find both the cylinder axis and power with a few easy-to-learn maneuvers. We owe it our gratitude for what it can do for us. **It should be loved, not feared!**

Positioning the Patient

Prior to positioning the patient, clean the forehead rest and the back of the phoropter with an alcohol pad.

The phoropter will elevate slightly as it is being locked into position. After the phoropter is in place, check these four: distance/near convergence levers, the position of the pupils, the vertex distance, and the leveling bubble.

The **forehead rest** should be extended to its maximal length, with the patient being told, "I'll bring the machine to you." Extending the forehead rest prevents the patient from being too close to the phoropter lenses, possibly rubbing lashes against them. Bringing the phoropter toward the patient, rather than having the patient lean forward at the start, allows you to move the forehead rest (with the patient's head gently against it) to the proper position without the patient possibly leaning forward excessively.

Center each pupil in the viewing aperture by adjusting the **interpupillary distance (PD) knob**. Do so after making certain the distance/near convergence levers are in the wide position, with each pushed fully to the side. After the distance refraction is completed, if near vision is to be evaluated to determine the proper Add, the levers are then moved fully inward. This will position the phoropter lenses for the convergence that will occur with close reading.

The patient's working position should be such that the phoropter lenses are positioned at the anticipated position of the eyeglasses lenses, or the **glasses plane**. The **vertex distance** is the interval between the outer surface of the cornea and the inner surface of a correcting lens. This distance plays an important role in precise focusing onto the retina, especially with larger refractive errors.

Prior to beginning, check these four (in this order):

1. Distance/Near convergence levers
2. Position of pupils
3. Vertex distance
4. Leveling bubble

The patient's position is best adjusted by glancing around the side of the phoropter and turning the forehead adjustment knob until the patient's lashes are near, but not touching, the lenses. Alternatively, one can use the mirrors located at the sides of the phoropter. **When refraction of the right eye has been completed, it is good to recheck the patient's position once again before refracting the left eye.**

The **leveling bubble** must be adjusted so that it is centered. It is checked last because the bubble's position will change if the phoropter is moved. An exception to centering the leveling bubble occurs if the patient has a chronic head tilt, which will result in the glasses frames being tilted. In that situation, the phoropter should have a matching tilt.

Stand on the right side of the patient when refracting each eye. Remember to occlude the left eye when beginning the right eye's refraction, and conversely for the left eye's refraction. Prior to beginning the left eye's refraction, open its viewing aperture before occluding the right eye. If not done in this sequence, both eyes will be occluded momentarily, and some patients find this disconcerting.

Note

It is **not** necessary to have all of the **lights** off in the examining room when subjective refraction is being performed. Most modern projection charts have sufficient luminosity to permit some ambient light. The projection chart should be approximately 30 times as luminous as the ambient light.

Having dim illumination in the exam room allows the refractionist to see the numbers while changing power and axis.

It is preferable to have a consistent level of illumination during subjective refraction so that it is not a variable when comparing visual acuity from one visit to the next.

THE THREE TYPES OF REFRACTION

▶ **Manifest refraction**: A refraction without cycloplegic drops; it is also called a "dry" refraction.

▶ **Cycloplegic refraction**: A refraction done with cycloplegic drops given to dilate the pupils and prevent accommodation; it is also called a "wet" refraction.

▶ **Post-cycloplegic refraction**: A dry refraction performed on a visit at least several days after a wet refraction. The purpose is to see how much of the full cycloplegic refraction found on the previous visit can be tolerated.

THE FOUR STEPS OF SUBJECTIVE REFRACTION

Subjective refraction consists of **four sequential refinement steps** performed in the following order:
1. **Step 1: Sphere**
2. **Step 2: Cylinder axis**
3. **Step 3: Cylinder power**
4. **Step 4: Sphere**

The purpose of each of the four steps is to locate the correct **endpoint**. This is accomplished by moving first in larger, then smaller, increments in order to hone in on the endpoint for each step. The process is referred to as **refinement**. This method is similar to how an address can be located on a map, first finding the city, then neighborhood, then street, and then house.

During each of the four steps, the patient is given a series of choices and asked to make a comparison, letting you know which of the two choices you are showing is clearer, or whether they appear to be the same in clarity.

There are two systems used for determining a patient's refractive error: the **plus cylinder method** and the **minus cylinder method**. They are two different ways of measuring the same thing, just like inches and meters. Most refractionists work in one of the methods exclusively, depending on their training. Where the methods differ, they are discussed separately with **black tabs** designating plus cylinder pages and **red tabs** designating minus cylinder pages.

Refining cylinder axis always precedes refinement of cylinder power. The correct axis can be located before power is refined, but the correct power can only be determined at the correct axis.

The **right eye** should **always** be refracted **first** and recorded **first**. This will prevent the prescription being written with the eyes reversed (and for the rest of the eye examination, the right eye should be evaluated first to prevent notation error).

Work with the smallest line on the acuity chart that is successfully read. This allows the patient to make the finest discrimination between the choices presented. As the refraction progresses, the line is lowered periodically. Improvement in **visual acuity** confirms the refraction is moving in the right direction.

Step 1: Sphere

The **large sphere power dial** at the side of the phoropter is used to show the patient a series of **two choices** to compare. The patient is asked to compare the two and tell you **which is more clear**, or that they appear the same in clarity.

- ▸ With the sphere power to be refined in place, choices are given in the plus and minus direction, changing the sphere based on the patient's preferences.

- ▸ Begin with choices 0.50-diopter apart before further refining in 0.25-diopter increments. If the patient has poor vision, or has difficulty making fine discriminations, give choices in larger increments.

- ▸ **Always checking in the plus direction first** is helpful in trying to avoid stimulating accommodation, and it keeps the method consistent. Whether in the plus or minus range, pulling down is adding plus power and pushing up is adding minus power.

Sphere is refined in Steps 1 and 4:

◆ Step 1 (in an eye with astigmatism) places the circle of least confusion, the blur circle, onto the retina.

◆ Step 4 (after the astigmatism has been corrected in Steps 2 and 3) places the focal point onto the retina.

Endpoint is the spherical lens that is reported by the patient to yield **the clearest view** of the letters on the acuity chart. If the patient reports the clarity between two choices to be **the same**, **always favor less minus**. (See *Over-Minusing* on page 60.)

Note

If the patient has no astigmatism, Step 1 places the focal point onto the retina; it is the same as Step 4.

Step 2: Cylinder Axis—Plus Cylinder Method

Locating the cylinder axis precedes determining the cylinder power. The correct axis will be found with the not yet refined (incorrect) cylinder power. Cylinder power will not be correct if measured at the wrong axis.

The **JCC** is used to refine the cylinder axis. It **leads** and **determines how the axis knob is turned**. After it is lowered into position, the thumb and forefinger are placed on top of the flip dials. The JCC is then turned clockwise until it clicks into position with the **white and red dots on either side of the axis arrow**.

The JCC is now **straddling the axis**.

The working axis is identified by two arrows 180 degrees apart on the large axis "clock," which has a mark every 5 degrees. There are corresponding axis arrows 180 degrees apart beneath the JCC with a mark every 15 degrees.

To avoid confusion, pick one of the arrows behind the JCC and work only with it and the dots surrounding it. The set most easily viewed should be used.

The JCC dial is then flipped, thereby giving a first and second choice to compare. The patient indicates which of the two choices can be seen more clearly. It is most efficient to always flip the dial in the same direction, even when repeating a pair of choices.

When the patient indicates which position of the JCC is clearer, **the axis is rotated in the direction of the white dot** for that choice (i.e., **"follow the white"**; Figure 2-2).

Begin with larger steps, typically 10-degree changes. Then, as the correct axis is approached, make 5-degree shifts. If initially there is significant uncertainty about axis location, you can move in 15-degree steps.

Reminder: The JCC—Dr. Jackson—leads and the cylinder axis knob follows its instructions.

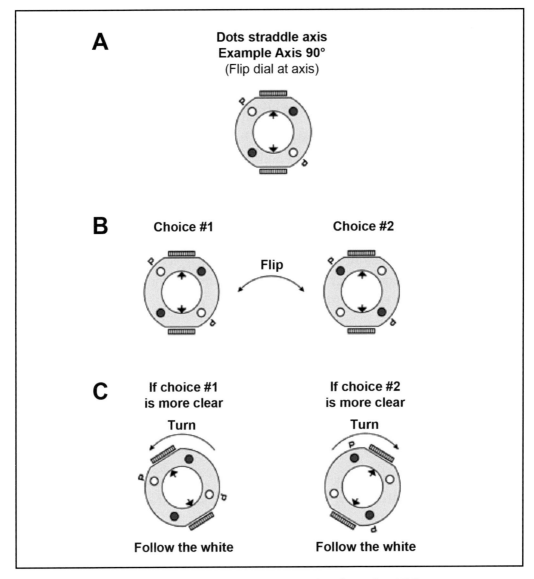

Figure 2-2. Refining the PLUS CYLINDER AXIS using the JCC.

   A. Position the JCC so that the red and white dots are "straddling the axis" to be refined (i.e., one dot on each side of the axis arrow).

   B. Look at one axis arrow and the set of dots surrounding it. Flip the cross cylinder to give the patient two choices, asking which is more clear.

   C. Rotate the axis in the direction of the white dot: FOLLOW THE WHITE.

If choice 1 is clearer, the white dot is on the left; turn the axis to the left.

If choice 2 is clearer, the white dot is on the right; turn the axis to the right.

The correct cylinder axis has been located when the cross cylinder is flipped and the patient responds that the two choices are "the same" in clarity.

The higher the cylinder power, the easier it is to locate the axis. If, in Step 3, cylinder power increases significantly, go back and recheck the axis (and then power again.)

Endpoint when refining cylinder axis: The two choices given to the patient are reported to be **the same** in clarity. At this point, **the correct axis is being bracketed**.

As cylinder axis refinement is concluding, a patient may go back and forth between two 5-degrees–apart choices, not responding "the same" for either choice. This indicates the axis is somewhere between the two choices. In this situation, it is fine to select the choice closer to 90 or 180 degrees as the endpoint (or the one closer to the axis in the patient's current glasses).

Note

When positioning the JCC in front of the patient's eye with **the axis straddled**, let the patient know that **the letters on the acuity chart will become more blurred**. Although neither of the choices you are giving for comparison is completely clear, you want to know which is **more** clear.

It may be necessary to move up one line on the acuity chart for the patient to see the letters well enough to compare the choices given.

Remember to return to a smaller line for Step 3.

Step 2: Cylinder Axis—Minus Cylinder Method

Locating the cylinder axis precedes determining the cylinder power. The correct axis will be found with the not yet refined (incorrect) cylinder power. Cylinder power will not be correct if measured at the wrong axis.

The **JCC** is used to refine the cylinder axis. It **leads** and **determines how the axis knob is turned**. After it is lowered into position, the thumb and forefinger are placed on top of the flip dials. The JCC is then turned clockwise until it clicks into position with **the white and red dots on either side of the axis arrow.**

The JCC is now **straddling the axis.**

The working axis is identified by two arrows 180 degrees apart on the large axis "clock," which has a mark every 5 degrees. There are corresponding axis arrows 180 degrees apart beneath the JCC with a mark every 15 degrees.

To avoid confusion, pick one of the arrows behind the JCC and work only with it and the dots surrounding it. The set most easily viewed should be used.

The JCC dial is then flipped, thereby giving a first and second choice to compare. The patient indicates which of the two choices can be seen more clearly. It is most efficient to always flip the dial in the same direction, even when repeating a pair of choices.

When the patient indicates which position of the JCC is clearer, **the axis is rotated in the direction of the red dot** for that choice (i.e., **"follow the red"**; Figure 2-3).

Begin with larger steps, typically 10-degree changes. Then, as the correct axis is approached, make 5-degree shifts. If initially there is significant uncertainty about axis location, you can move in 15-degree steps.

Reminder: The JCC—Dr. Jackson—leads and the cylinder axis knob follows its instructions.

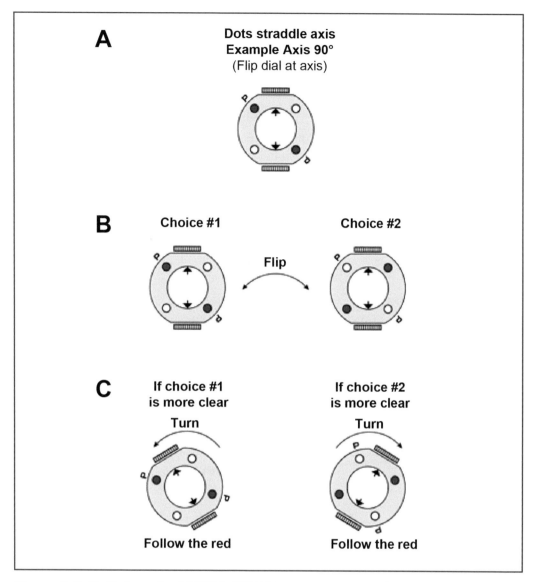

Figure 2-3. Refining the MINUS CYLINDER AXIS using the JCC.

   A. Position the JCC so that the red and white dots are "straddling the axis" to be refined (i.e., one dot on each side of the axis arrow).

   B. Look at one axis arrow and the set of dots surrounding it. Flip the cross cylinder to give the patient two choices, asking which is more clear.

   C. Rotate the axis in the direction of the red dot: FOLLOW THE RED.

If choice 1 is clearer, the red dot is on the left; turn the axis to the left.

If choice 2 is clearer, the red dot is on the right; turn the axis to the right.

The correct cylinder axis has been located when the cross cylinder is flipped and the patient responds that the two choices are "the same" in clarity.

The higher the cylinder power, the easier it is to locate the axis. If, in Step 3, cylinder power increases significantly, go back and recheck the axis (and then power again.)

Endpoint when refining cylinder axis: The two choices given to the patient are reported to be **the same** in clarity. At this point, **the correct axis is being bracketed**.

As cylinder axis refinement is concluding, a patient may go back and forth between two 5-degrees–apart choices, not responding "the same" for either choice. This indicates the axis is somewhere between the two choices. In this situation, it is fine to select the choice closer to 90 or 180 degrees as the endpoint (or the one closer to the axis in the patient's current glasses).

Note

When positioning the JCC in front of the patient's eye with **the axis straddled**, let the patient know that **the letters on the acuity chart will become more blurred**. Although neither of the choices you are giving for comparison is completely clear, you want to know which is **more** clear.

It may be necessary to move up one line on the acuity chart for the patient to see the letters well enough to compare the choices given.

Remember to return to a smaller line for Step 3.

Step 3: Cylinder Power—Plus Cylinder Method

The **JCC** is used to refine the cylinder power. It **leads** and **determines how the cylinder power knob is turned**. Both flip dials are again held to rotate the JCC clockwise until it clicks into place when **the red or white dot is aligned with the axis** determined in Step 2 (Figure 2-4).

White = Add cylinder power
Red = Subtract cylinder power

The JCC is now **on axis**; a dot overlies the arrow.

Choices are given by flipping the JCC, and the patient indicates which of the two choices you have shown is clearer. It is most efficient to always flip the dial in the same direction, even when repeating a pair of choices. If it was necessary to move up one line on the acuity chart for Step 2, return to the previous line to begin Step 3; acuity is better with the JCC on axis than when it is straddling the axis.

If the patient responds that the letters appear to be more clear when **the white dot is positioned on axis, then plus cylinder power is added** (i.e., white = add).

If the letters are more clear **when the red dot is positioned on axis, then plus cylinder power is subtracted** (i.e., red = subtract).

Cylinder power is usually modified by 0.25-diopter changes from the start.

> **Reminder:** The JCC—Dr. Jackson—leads and the cylinder axis knob follows its instructions.

During the process of refining cylinder power, an **adjustment to spherical power** must be made whenever the cylinder power has been modified by 0.50 diopter. The adjustment is necessary to reposition the circle of least confusion onto the retina.

Endpoint when refining cylinder power: The two choices given the patient are **the same** in clarity. At this point, **the correct cylinder power is being bracketed**.

As cylinder power refinement is concluding, a patient may go back and forth between two 0.25-diopter–apart choices, not responding "the same" for either choice. This indicates the power is somewhere between the two choices. In this situation, it is fine to select the choice with less cylinder power as the endpoint.

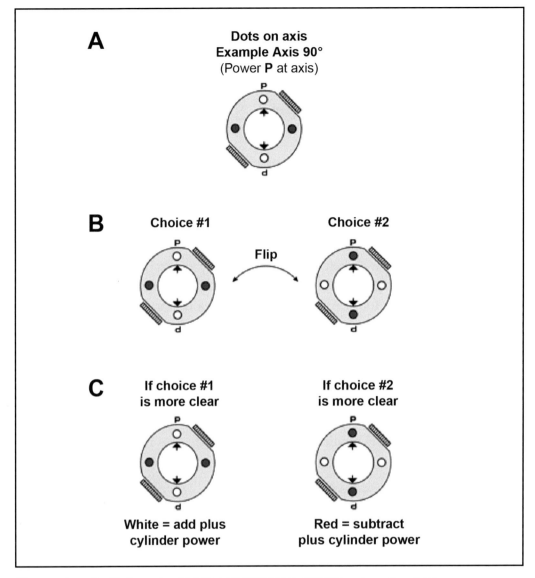

Figure 2-4. Refining the PLUS CYLINDER POWER using the JCC.

   A. Turn the JCC clockwise so that the red or white dot is "on axis" (i.e., aligned with the axis determined by the previous step).

   B. Flip the cross cylinder to give the patient two choices, asking which is more clear.

   C. Add or subtract cylinder power: WHITE = ADD; RED = SUTRACT.

If choice 1 is clearer, the white dot is chosen; add plus cylinder power.

If choice 2 is clearer, the red dot is chosen; subtract plus cylinder power. (See *The Adjustment Within Step 3* on page 45.)

The correct cylinder power has been determined when the cross cylinder is flipped and the patient responds that the two choices are "the same" in clarity.

Step 3: Cylinder Power—Minus Cylinder Method

The **JCC** is used to refine the cylinder power. It **leads** and **determines how the cylinder power knob is turned**. Both flip dials are again held

Red = Add cylinder power

White = Subtract cylinder power

to rotate the JCC clockwise until it clicks into place when **the red or white dot is aligned with the axis** determined in Step 2 (Figure 2-5).

The JCC is now **on axis**; a dot overlies the arrow.

Choices are given by flipping the JCC, and the patient indicates which of the two choices you have shown is clearer. It is most efficient to always flip the dial in the same direction, even when repeating a pair of choices. If it was necessary to move up one line on the acuity chart for Step 2, return to the previous line to begin Step 3; acuity is better with the JCC on axis than when it is straddling the axis.

If the patient responds that the letters appear to be more clear **when the red dot is positioned on axis, then minus cylinder power is added** (i.e., red = add).

If the letters are more clear **when the white dot is positioned on axis, then minus cylinder power is subtracted** (i.e., white = subtract).

Cylinder power is usually modified by 0.25-diopter changes from the start.

> **Reminder:** The JCC—Dr. Jackson—leads and the cylinder axis knob follows its instructions.

During the process of refining the cylinder power, an **adjustment to spherical power** must be made whenever the cylinder power has been modified by 0.50 diopter. The adjustment is necessary to reposition the circle of least confusion onto the retina.

Endpoint when refining cylinder power: The two choices given the patient are **the same** in clarity. At this point, **the correct cylinder power is being bracketed**.

As cylinder power refinement is concluding, a patient may go back and forth between two 0.25-diopter–apart choices, not responding "the same" for either choice. This indicates the power is somewhere between the two choices. In this situation, it is fine to select the choice with less cylinder power as the endpoint.

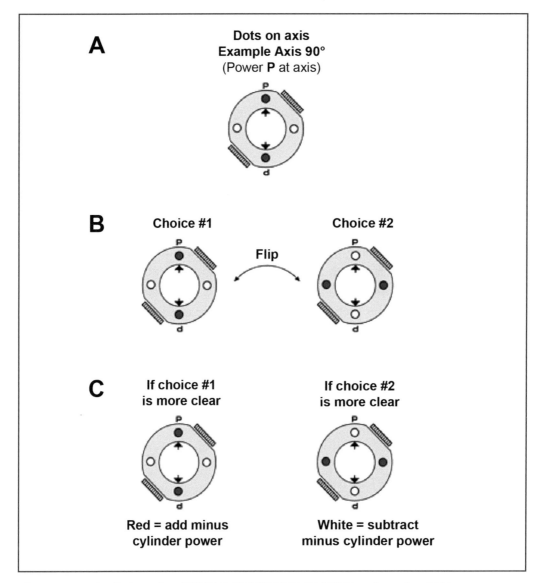

Figure 2-5. Refining the MINUS CYLINDER POWER using the JCC.

 A. Turn the JCC clockwise so that the red or white dot is "on axis" (i.e., aligned with the axis determined by the previous step).

 B. Flip the cross cylinder to give the patient two choices, asking which is more clear.

 C. Add or subtract cylinder power: RED = ADD; WHITE = SUBTRACT.

If choice 1 is clearer, the red dot is chosen; add minus cylinder power.

If choice 2 is clearer, the white dot is chosen; subtract minus cylinder power. (See *The Adjustment Within Step 3* on page 45.)

The correct cylinder power has been determined when the cross cylinder is flipped and the patient responds that the two choices are "the same" in clarity.

THE ADJUSTMENT WITHIN STEP 3

When refining cylinder power, an **adjustment to the spherical power** found in Step 1 must be made for every 0.50-diopter change in **cylinder power**. The adjustment is made whenever 0.50 diopter of cylinder power is added or subtracted. The adjustment is necessary to reposition the circle of least confusion, the blur circle, onto the retina. This enables the patient to make the best discriminations going forward. The **spherical equivalent** is used to make the adjustment.

The conoid of Sturm is represented by the interval of Sturm in Figures 2-6 through 2-9.

Optically:

- A change in cylinder power moves one focal line—the one parallel to the axis.

- A change in sphere power moves the conoid of Sturm—both focal lines.

The Adjustment Within Step 3: Plus Cylinder Method

An adjustment to the spherical power (determined in Step 1) must be made for every 0.50-diopter change in cylinder power. The adjustment is necessary to reposition the blur circle onto the retina, which will then enable the patient to make the best discriminations going forward. The spherical equivalent is used to make the adjustment.

The Rule When Adding Plus Cylinder Power

For every 0.50 diopter of plus cylinder power added, remove 0.25 diopter of plus sphere power.

Optically, the following is occurring (Figure 2-6):

 A. The circle of least confusion (the blur circle) has been placed on the retina in Step 1. It is always dioptrically midway between the two focal lines.

 B. **0.50 of plus cylinder power is added at 90 degrees.** A cylinder affects the focal line that is parallel to its axis. The addition of plus cylinder power has moved the vertical focal line forward and the conoid of Sturm is collapsing. The blur circle has become smaller and has moved to the left, midway between the two focal lines.

 C. **The adjustment: 0.25 of plus spherical power is removed.** The spherical lens change has moved both focal lines posteriorly, and the blur circle is located at its mid-position. This adjustment has repositioned the blur circle onto the retina.

 D. The previous two steps are repeated as necessary until the two focal lines meet. When they meet, the conoid of Sturm is fully collapsed and only a focal point remains. (The position of the focal point is refined in Step 4.)

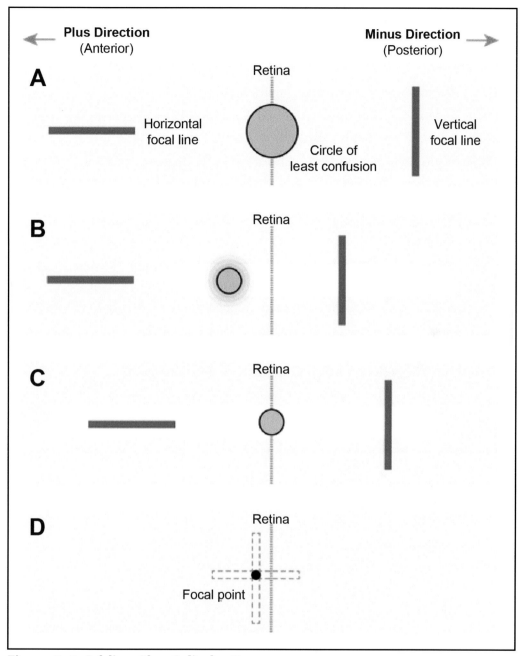

Figure 2-6. Adding Plus Cylinder Power.

The Rule When Subtracting Plus Cylinder Power

For every 0.50 diopter of plus cylinder power removed, add 0.25 diopter of plus sphere power.

Optically, the following is occurring (Figure 2-7):

A. The circle of least confusion (the blur circle) has been placed on the retina in Step 1. It is always dioptrically midway between the two focal lines.

B. **0.50 of plus cylinder power is subtracted at 90 degrees.** A cylinder affects the focal line that is parallel to its axis. The subtraction of plus cylinder power has moved the vertical focal line posteriorly and the conoid of Sturm is collapsing. The blur circle has become smaller and moved to the right, midway between the two focal lines.

C. **The adjustment: 0.25 of plus spherical power is added.** The spherical lens change has moved both focal lines anteriorly, and the blur circle is located at its mid-position. This adjustment has repositioned the blur circle onto the retina.

D. The previous two steps are repeated as necessary until the two focal lines meet. When they meet, the conoid of Sturm is fully collapsed and only a focal point remains. (The position of the focal point is refined in Step 4.)

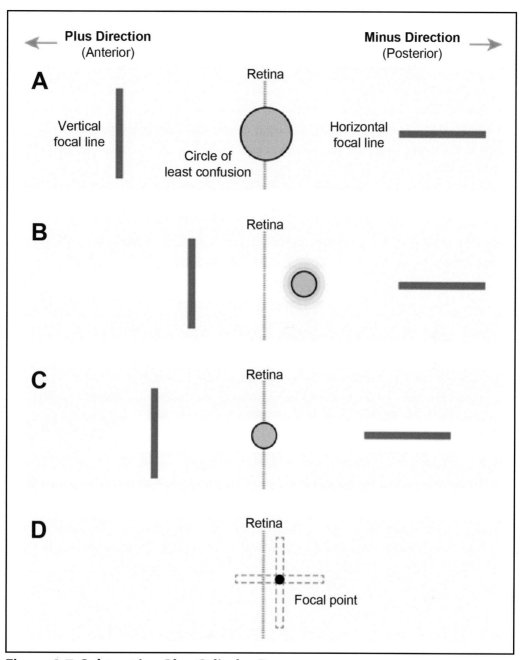

Figure 2-7. Subtracting Plus Cylinder Power.

The Adjustment Within Step 3: Minus Cylinder Method

An adjustment to the **spherical power** (determined in Step 1) must be made for every 0.50-diopter change in **cylinder power**. The adjustment is necessary to reposition the blur circle onto the retina, which will then enable the patient to make the best discriminations going forward. The spherical equivalent is used to make the adjustment.

The Rule When Adding Minus Cylinder Power

For every 0.50 diopter of minus cylinder power added, remove 0.25 diopter of minus sphere power.

Optically, the following is occurring (Figure 2-8):

A. The circle of least confusion (the blur circle) has been placed on the retina in Step 1. It is always dioptrically midway between the two focal lines.

B. **0.50 of minus cylinder power is added at 90 degrees.** A cylinder affects the focal line that is parallel to its axis. The addition of minus cylinder power has moved the vertical focal line posteriorly and the conoid of Sturm is collapsing. The blur circle has become smaller and moved to the right, midway between the two focal lines.

C. **The adjustment: 0.25 of minus spherical power is removed.** The spherical lens change has moved both focal lines anteriorly, and the blur circle is located at its mid-position. This adjustment has repositioned the blur circle onto the retina.

D. The previous two steps are repeated as necessary until the two focal lines meet. When they meet, the conoid of Sturm is fully collapsed and only a focal point remains. (The position of the focal point is refined in Step 4.)

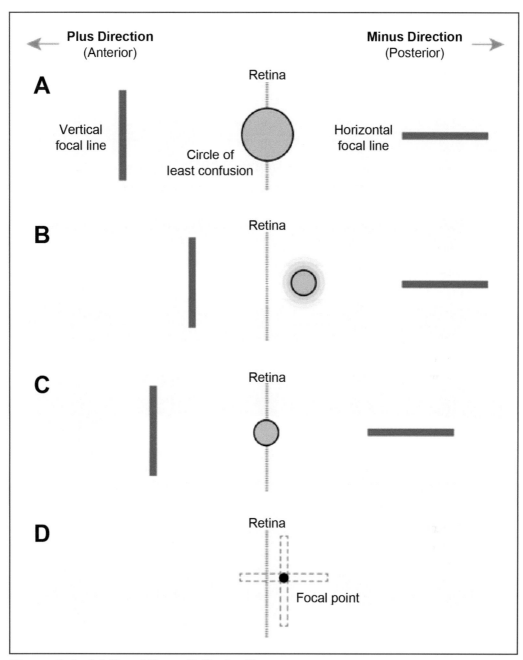

Figure 2-8. Adding Minus Cylinder Power.

The Rule When Subtracting Minus Cylinder Power

For every 0.50 diopter of minus cylinder power removed, add 0.25 diopter of minus sphere power.

Optically, the following is occurring (Figure 2-9):

A. The circle of least confusion (the blur circle) has been placed on the retina in Step 1. It is always dioptrically midway between the two focal lines.

B. **0.50 of minus cylinder power is subtracted at 90 degrees.** A cylinder affects the focal line that is parallel to its axis. The subtraction of minus cylinder power has moved the vertical focal line forward and the conoid of Sturm is collapsing. The blur circle has become smaller and has moved to the left, midway between the two focal lines.

C. **The adjustment: 0.25 of minus spherical power is added.** The spherical lens change has moved both focal lines posteriorly, and the blur circle is located at its mid-position. This adjustment has repositioned the blur circle onto the retina.

D. The above two steps are repeated as necessary until the two focal lines meet. When they meet, the conoid of Sturm is fully collapsed and only a focal point remains. (The position of the focal point is refined in Step 4.)

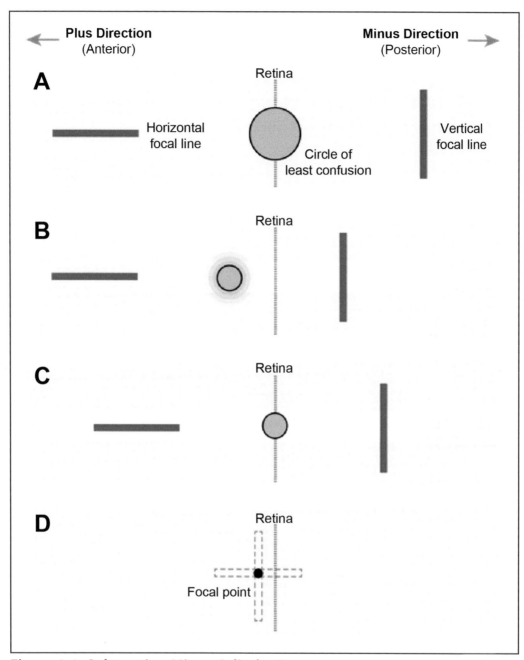

Figure 2-9. Subtracting Minus Cylinder Power.

An **airplane luggage analogy** may be helpful when performing the adjustment within Step 3 (Figures 2-10 and 2-11).

- ▸ **A small suitcase represents one click of the "small" cylinder power knob.**
- ▸ **A large suitcase represents one click of the "large" sphere power dial.**
- ▸ Two small suitcases equal one large suitcase.
- ▸ Within each method, the sphere sign is the same as the cylinder sign.

The cargo hold must be filled to capacity.

- ▸ **If two small suitcases are added, one large suitcase must be removed.**
- ▸ **If two small suitcases are removed, one large suitcase must be added.**

A 2:1 Ratio for the Adjustment:

- ◆ 2 little (cylinder knob clicks) = 1 big (sphere dial click)

Note

For Step 3, remember to **return to a smaller line** if a larger one was used during axis refinement in Step 2.

If the cylinder power increases significantly in Step 3, recheck the axis (and then power again). The greater the cylinder power, the easier it is to locate the correct axis.

Steps 2 and 3 collapse the conoid of Sturm to a single focal point.

Step 4 places the focal point onto the retina.

If there is no astigmatism, Step 1 placed the focal point onto the retina.

If there is astigmatism, Step 1 placed the blur circle onto the retina.

The JCC is now removed—it has done its job!

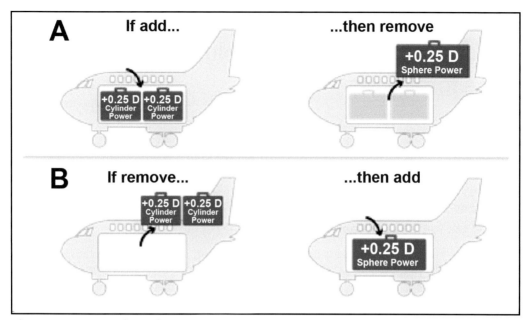

Figure 2-10. Airplane luggage analogy—Plus Cylinder Method.

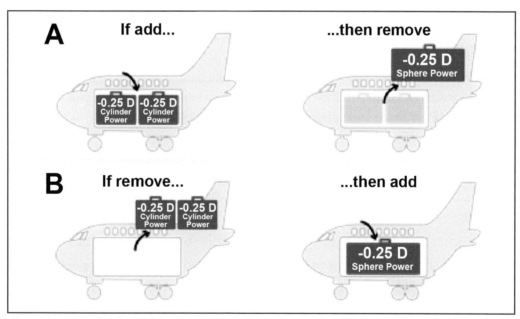

Figure 2-11. Airplane luggage analogy—Minus Cylinder Method.

At the conclusion of Steps 2 and 3, the astigmatism has been corrected and the blur circle is transformed into a focal point.

Step 4: Sphere

As in Step 1, the **large sphere power dial** at the side of the phoropter is used to show the patient a series of **two choices** to compare. The patient is asked to compare the two and tell you **which is more clear**, or that they appear the same in clarity.

▶ Choices are given in the plus and minus direction, changing the sphere based on the patient's preferences.

▶ Begin with choices 0.50-diopter apart before further refining in 0.25-diopter increments. If the patient has poor vision or has difficulty making fine discriminations, give choices in larger increments.

▶ **Always checking in the plus direction first** is helpful in trying to avoid stimulating accommodation, and it keeps the method consistent. Whether in the plus or minus range, pulling down is adding plus power, pushing up is adding minus power.

Endpoint: the spherical lens that is reported by the patient to yield **the clearest** view of the letters on the acuity chart. If the patient says the clarity between two choices is **the same, always favor less minus**. (See *Over-Minusing* on page 60.)

Note

The spherical refinement in Step 4 places the **focal point onto the retina**.

If the sphere changes significantly during this step, repeat Steps 3 and 4.

During Step 4, **additional tests** can be used to check for over-minusing. (See *Over-Minusing* on page 60.)

(See *Instructing the Patient* on page 57, *Sixteen Tips for Accurate Subjective Refraction Results* on page 63, and Chapter 3 for more detail and tips for performing the Four Steps of Subjective Refraction.)

To find if cylinder is present when starting de novo, see Tip 9 on page 64.

(See *Astigmatism Case 3* on page 85 to learn what to do when, in Step 3, cylinder power has been reduced to .00 and the patient then chooses less cylinder power.)

Instructing the Patient

The efficiency and final result of subjective refraction can be maximized by guiding the patient through the process with the proper instructions. There is no one right way to do this, and each refractionist will arrive at a preferred method.

Just before having the patient look through the phoroptor or trial frame, explain that you are now going to perform a refraction, the measurement to determine the optimal glasses prescription, and the best visual acuity. Then proceed with instructing the patient:

"I'm going to give you some choices. I will show you sets of two lenses to compare, and I want you to tell me which is more clear, the first way or the second way. If they seem 'about the same,' that is always a good answer."

After the initial instructions, describing the choice for the patient as "**the first way or the second way**" can be abbreviated to "**first or second**," "**number one or number two**," or "**one or two**." Since you are always giving the patient a choice between two lenses for comparison, using the numbers "one" and "two" is all that is necessary and has the element of simplicity.

Some refractionists prefer to number subsequent choices "three or four," "five or six," "seven or eight," etc. Using the **additional numbers** can be helpful for the occasional patient who continually responds, for example, "two," and seems to be moving away from the correct endpoint. On the other hand, if a patient were to respond, "I think I liked number three better than number six," it can create some confusion.

Each lens and its number should be given to the patient **simultaneously**. Present the two lenses for comparison in a **smooth, consecutive** fashion. The speed should be **fairly rapid**, as the comparison is a test of first impression. Repeat the choices if the patient requests, if the patient pauses, if the lenses are not presented smoothly, or if the lens and number are not presented simultaneously.

It is good to **avoid asking which choice is "better"** because letters becoming "smaller and darker" can look better to the patient. "Smaller and darker" is an indication of over-minusing. (See *Over-Minusing* on page 60.) We should ask, **"Which is more clear...?"**

It is also good to avoid the potential confusion of asking the patient, "Which is better, this one or that one?"
because if "that one" is the second choice shown, it is
technically both "that one" and "this one."

The acuity chart can project a single letter, a single line,
or multiple lines. Refractionists differ in their preferred presentation. Many simply
project a single line, moving down the chart in that manner. Some ask patients to
concentrate on a particular letter when a single line is shown, and patients will sometimes adopt this strategy on their own. Other refractionists prefer to have the patient
view round rather than square letters, believing it will be helpful when correcting
astigmatism.

No Conversation

To be most efficient, it is generally best to steer the patient toward
responding only with a number or "same."

A "**no conversation**" approach often is a big help in making the process go smoothly,
quickly, and correctly. This is in contrast to taking a medical history, when it is often
beneficial to expand the narrative.

If asked more open-ended questions such as, "Which do you like?" or "Is this better?"
the patient may want to describe various aspects of what is seen. A descriptive response
tends to slow the process down considerably and is usually not helpful. Even a first and
second choice of "this one" or "that one" can create confusion because if the patient
says "this one," that may indicate the first or second choice!

This is why numbers are used.

Managing Pauses

It is important to properly manage the pauses that can often occur after the patient
has been shown two choices to compare. A pause is usually due to uncertainty on the
patient's part, and it is best not to simply wait for a response.

Once you detect the pause, immediately show the patient the choices once again,
saying, "**Let me show you again.**" Giving the choices a second time often helps the
patient decide, and greatly expedites the refraction. Many times, it is the patient who
will request you give the choices again!

Subjective refraction is a **test of first impression**, and it works best when the patient does not "study" the choices. If there is continued uncertainty on the patient's part, it suggests the two choices are about the same. Thus, the refinement is at or near the endpoint.

Alternatively, pauses may indicate the differences shown are too small for the patient to make distinctions, and it is then necessary to move to larger increments of change.

Notes on "About the Same"

If the patient says the two choices you have given are "**the same**" or "**about the same**":

When completing the refinement of spherical power (Steps 1 and 4), if there is not a clear between two lenses, the endpoint is the less minus of the two choices. This prevents over-minusing.

When locating cylinder axis with the JCC (Step 2), you have arrived at the correct endpoint. Neither to the left nor to the right of the current axis is clearer. **Each choice is moving equally away from the now correct axis**; thus, they are "the same."

When measuring cylinder power with the JCC (Step 3), you have arrived at the correct endpoint. Neither the addition nor the subtraction of power is clearer. **Each choice is moving equally away from the now correct power**; thus, they are "the same."

Thus, "about the same" is music to the ears of a refractionist, as it concludes Steps 2 and 3—and also marks the end of Steps 1 and 4, indicating that the less minus choice is the end point.

When Straddling the Axis

When beginning the refinement of the patient's astigmatism correction (Step 2), the JCC is positioned to straddle the axis. When the JCC is placed in this position, the patient will notice that the vision is less clear than it was at the end of Step 1. It is therefore helpful to tell the patient, before moving the cross cylinder into place, that **you will be making things a little more blurred**. During the testing, the patient can be told, "**Neither of these choices will be perfect, but tell me which one is clearer.**"

Note

Because of the slight blurring induced at the beginning of this step, **it is sometimes necessary to move one line higher on the Snellen chart** so that you are working with a line the patient can read. Once the cross cylinder has been moved into place, determine whether the patient can still read the line you were using at the end of Step 1. If it cannot be read, move one line higher.

Remember to move back to a lower Snellen line when, in Step 3, the cross cylinder is positioned on axis.

Over-Minusing

If, at the conclusion of a refraction, the measurement contains **more minus spherical correction than the true refractive error**, the patient has been "**over-minused**."

Over-minusing is the result of the patient **accommodating during the refraction**. When the patient is accommodating, more internal plus spherical power is added to the eye. Thus, externally, additional minus spherical power is chosen to offset it. The extra minus is not correcting the basic refractive error; it is offsetting the accommodation.

If a patient were to be prescribed the over-minused measurement, the patient would need to continually accommodate for the focal point to remain on the retina when looking in the distance. This chronic accommodative effort can cause **eye fatigue**. In addition, it would leave less accommodation available for focusing at near, likely resulting in a complaint of eye strain with reading.

The following can be seen in a patient who has been over-minused:

▶ Eye strain from excessive accommodation

▶ The need for an "early" bifocal because accommodation has been "used up," off-setting the extra minus

▶ Minification of images viewed

▶ An artificial increase in measured plus cylinder power and artificial decrease in measured minus cylinder power (See *Astigmatism Case 4* on page 86.)

There are four ways to avoid over-minusing during subjective refraction: **instructing the patient properly, cycloplegia, fogging techniques, and the duochrome test. The first two are the most commonly used.**

1. If subjective refraction is performed without cycloplegia, it is important to **instruct the patient properly** to prevent over-minusing when measuring the sphere. During Steps 1 and 4, the patient should be told, "**Compare clarity. If one of the choices makes the letters smaller and darker, ignore that.**" The smaller and darker phenomenon results from a reverse Galilean telescope effect, and it is a sign of over-minusing. The reason this instruction needs to be emphasized is that the patient may like the appearance of the smaller and darker letters, thus it is best to avoid asking which choice is "better."

2. A **cycloplegic refraction** eliminates the concern about over-minusing as the patient is unable to accommodate.

3. **Fogging techniques** blur vision by adding plus sphere power. There are several ways this can be done. A simple and efficient method is as follows. At the end of Step 4, if there is concern about over-minusing, plus sphere power is added until the existing line of best acuity becomes blurred. Three-quarters of a diopter will usually achieve this. Plus sphere power is then removed in 0.25-diopter steps, stopping as soon as the previous line of best acuity is read clearly. At that sphere power, the patient is not over-minused.

   Fogging can be performed monocularly or binocularly. The latter method, termed **binocular balancing**, makes certain the two eyes have been fogged equally. The prism dials of the phoropter can be used to allow both eyes to view the acuity chart at the same time with separate images for comparison. **A line on the acuity chart is split vertically into separate images, one for each eye, by the prisms. The eyes are then fogged equally. Plus power is then removed simultaneously and equally from each eye, arriving at an endpoint as described for monocular fogging.**

4. The **duochrome test** utilizes the differing wavelengths of colors and the chromatic aberration within the eye. Letters on the red and green halves of the screen should appear equally clear. If they do not, this indicates that additional plus or minus spherical power is needed. If the **red side** of the screen appears to the patient to be clearer, more **minus power** is needed. If the **green side** of the screen is clearer, the eye is **over-minused** and more **plus power** is necessary.

   Remember **Red Add Minus, Green Add Plus** with the mnemonic **RAMGAP**.

   The duochrome test will not be helpful if the patient's visual acuity is worse than 20/30. Also, it is subject to error if the patient is accommodating.

Encouragement

Comparing visual acuity from visit to visit is an integral part of monitoring the status of a patient's medical eye problem (e.g., for age-related macular degeneration or diabetic macular edema). To make proper comparisons from visit to visit, the amount of effort the patient makes when reading the letters on the acuity chart must be kept as consistent as possible. **It is not unusual for a patient to state that a line is too difficult to read, but then be able to read it when encouraged.**

Phrases such as "**Give it a try**" or "**Do the best you can**" are very helpful in this regard.

It is preferable to **avoid telling the patient to "guess"** as it can give the patient an improper impression of the importance of determining visual acuity.

Three Patient Concerns

There are three patient concerns, often expressed, during the process of subjective refraction:

1. The patient feels the choices are being given **too fast.**

2. The patient is worried about the choices **not being consistent**, thus leading to a wrong prescription.

3. The patient is not naming the letters correctly, thus **not getting the answers "right."**

The following are possible ways to alleviate these patient apprehensions:

1. If the patient feels the choices are being presented too fast, it is helpful to explain that the comparison of lenses in subjective refraction is a **test of first impression.** It works best if the choices are not studied or "worked on." Understanding this often results in the patient being more relaxed through the process.

2. A patient who is concerned about consistency is usually reassured if you explain, **"That is for me to worry about. You are doing fine."**

3. The concern about getting **"the right answer"** is understandable. Isn't that what we all tried to do in school? So, what should you do if the patient asks, "Is that a B?" As a general rule, **there is no need to ever tell the patient what the letter is.**

One way to respond is, **"You know, we are sworn to secrecy."** Patients usually enjoy the humor, and it is a way of indicating that the purpose of the test is not to get every letter right. The purpose of the test is to determine the level of the patient's visual acuity. From that perspective, the patient can be told, **"This is a test that everyone passes."** In fact, **everyone's score is perfect**. The responses have been perfect because the **level of visual acuity has been determined**!

Sixteen Tips for Accurate Subjective Refraction Results

1. **Move through the four steps expeditiously.** This makes the process more efficient, more precise, and easier for the patient and the examiner. Comparing different lenses during subjective refraction is a **test of first impression**. A good rule of thumb is to not wait for a delayed response (i.e., have a **"no pauses" policy**). A pause is the result of the patient being uncertain which of the two lenses is better. Therefore, once a pause occurs, show the choice again and remind the patient that "**the same**" is always a good answer. If there is still a pause upon reshowing, consider it identical to a response of "the same." Keep moving!

2. When initially measuring a patient's visual acuity, there is **no need to start with the larger letters** on the visual acuity chart unless you have an indication that visual acuity is reduced. The goal is to determine the smallest line the patient can read, and you want to get there as efficiently as possible.

3. During subjective refraction, **work with the smallest line that the patient can read, going further down as acuity is improving**. The patient is able to make finer discriminations on the smaller lines.

4. Watch to make sure the patient is **not squinting** as this will give an unwanted pinhole effect.

5. Run through the sequence again **if there is a large change in any of the steps.**

6. When working with the JCC, while checking cylinder axis and power, there are two viewing strategies that can be employed **if the patient selects choice 1.** (If the patient chooses choice 2, one can directly visualize where the white and red dots are located.)

   If the patient says choice 1 was clearer, you can either **flip back** to the first choice and see where the dots are or **not flip back** but know that choice 1 was the opposite of what you are seeing now. The "not flip back" strategy saves one flip each time the patient chooses "number 1."

   One reasonable approach is for the novice refractionist to flip back to choice 1 if it is chosen in order to lessen the chance for confusion. With experience, that extra flip can be abandoned.

7. When refining sphere, two different methods may be employed with regard to **the first lens presented for the next set of choices.** The first lens shown can either be a **new lens** or the **lens the patient is currently looking through if that was the chosen lens from the previous set.**

Some refractionists feel it is important to always show the patient a new lens at the start of each set. Others find it is not necessary to do so. Using the lens already in place from the previous set of choices, if that was the chosen lens, does save an additional flip.

8. **If the patient has reduced vision due to an eye disease**, use large steps throughout. If it is available, a hand-held +/- 0.50 or +/- 1.00 diopter cross cylinder can be helpful.

9. **When starting a refraction de novo** (i.e., without prior retinoscopy, autorefraction, or old glasses), **it is necessary to determine if astigmatism is present**. (If one of these modalities is used and indicates sphere only, it is still necessary to check to see if there is astigmatism.) This requires an **extra step**, not part of the standard four, and can be considered Step 1a. It should be performed unless the patient is reading 20/20 crisply with a spherical correction.

There are two ways to do the extra step, with and without the JCC:

   i. **Using the JCC** (for plus and minus cylinder methods):
   - With **no cylinder power** dialed in, give the patient choices: **flip the white and red dot at 90/180 degrees**. If the choices appear "the same," then flip at **45/135 degrees**.
   - If the patient finds no difference during each set of comparisons, it can be concluded that no astigmatism is likely to be present.
   - If one of the choices is more clear, dial in 0.50 of cylinder power at that axis, adjust the sphere by 0.25 diopter, and **proceed with Step 2**.

   ii. **Not using the JCC** (for plus and minus cylinder methods):
   - Dial **0.50 of cylinder power** in and then out at these axes: 90, 180, 45, 135.
   - If none of the choices presented increase clarity, it can be concluded that no astigmatism is likely to be present.
   - If one of the choices is more clear, stop, keep it in place, adjust the sphere by 0.25 diopter, and **proceed with Step 2**.

10. **It is sometimes the case that a patient's subjective responses are inconsistent or unreliable.** In this situation, **do not let yourself get frustrated**, which is sometimes a tempting response. It is important to keep in mind that the patient came for eye care, not to cause you difficulty. When visual field testing yields unreliable responses, we glean whatever information we can from it and move on. An unreliable subjective refraction can be thought of in the same way.

Varying responses may be caused by a number of factors. The patient's **head can drift backward**, away from the forehead rest, resulting in a change in the **vertex distance**. Inconsistency can also result from **squinting**, which produces a pinhole effect, or from **staring**, causing corneal drying. **Medical eye problems** can also result in varying responses. Cataracts, macular edema, dry eye, age-related macular degeneration, and other conditions can cause vision to fluctuate.

If cylinder power increases significantly in Step 3, return to Step 2 to better refine the axis. The correct axis is more easily located with the increased cylinder power. Then continue with Step 3 once again.

Use visual acuity to make sure you are moving to the correct endpoint. If the acuity is worsening following the patient's choices, this indicates that the responses have been unreliable.

An earlier step in the sequence can be repeated. If this is done, continue from that step in the proper order. However, if you find the patient is not moving in the right direction, with acuity worsening instead of improving, **you can "break the sequence."** That is, you can **deviate from the normal sequence either during or after the four steps of subjective refraction**. You can make **larger jumps** in spherical power, cylinder axis, and cylinder power than you would normally, and the cylinder axis knob can even be turned freehand without use of the JCC.

It is important to understand that some patients can lead you to a very precise and repeatable endpoint, and others cannot.

If it seems that the patient's responses are not reliable enough to be helpful, it is important to **know when to quit**. In that situation, it should be noted on the patient's chart that the refraction resulted in a "**poor endpoint**."

11. During subjective refraction, we are giving choices and asking for the patient's preferences. However, **we as refractionists also have preferences**:

    - **Less minus in the sphere** to avoid over-minusing

    - **Less power in the cylinder** to make adjustment to the glasses easier for the patient

    - **Cylinder axis at 90 or 180 degrees** to lessen the chance that the patient will have tilting of viewed objects

    - **Oblique axes symmetrical, adding to 180 degrees**, which suggests that they are correct

    - **An Add that is age appropriate** (See *Four Points About Correcting Presbyopia With an Add* on page 16 and *Myopia Cases 3 and 4* on pages 78-79.)

12. If, during the spherical measurement, the patient keeps choosing lenses in the minus direction (this can be called the **minus march**) and then begins to progressively choose less minus, continue to allow the patient to move in the plus direction. This pattern can occur if accommodation is at first increasing, but subsequently relaxing, as the refraction proceeds. (See *Over-Minusing* on page 60 and *Myopia Case 1* on page 76.)

13. **If there is only 0.25 diopter of cylinder power**, it can be difficult to correctly position the axis.

14. **When refracting a child**, at the completion of the refraction, allow the patient to view the acuity chart binocularly. Add + 0.25 diopter of sphere to each eye and determine whether the child's ability to read the chart is unchanged. If it is unchanged, continue to remove minus binocularly until the visual acuity is affected. This additional step will **decrease the likelihood that a child will be over-minused** as a consequence of the very strong accommodative ability.

15. **When prescribing aphakic glasses, the vertex distance** must be specified. It is measured with a special caliper called a **distometer**. (See *Positioning the Patient* on page 30.)

16. It may be helpful to occasionally use **Halberg clips, supplemental cylinder power inserts, or the 0.0 power lens in the trial lens set**.

    A **Halberg clip** is placed over the lens in the patient's glasses. The clips are made to hold trial lenses that are placed in front of the lenses currently worn.

    A **supplemental cylinder power insert** is intended for use when the power of the patient's cylinder exceeds 6.00 diopters.

    The **0.0 power lens** can be helpful in several situations. It can be used in the trial frame to have consistency of lens additivity when one eye has a purely cylindrical correction. It can also be helpful as a "magic lens" for a patient whom you suspect of malingering or wanting to be like a sibling or friend who wears glasses.

BEFORE WRITING A GLASSES PRESCRIPTION

Show and Compare What You Plan to Give—Always!

This is an essential ending for the refraction process, and its importance cannot be overemphasized. Despite this, it is often omitted!

After the four steps of subjective refraction have been completed for each eye, **show** what you plan to give the patient binocularly. **It is essential that the patient be part of the decision-making process; the refractionist should not make the decision unilaterally.**

If the patient is currently wearing glasses, ask the patient to **compare** what has just been measured to the current glasses—the measurement in the phoropter versus the glasses. If the patient is **able to see more clearly** with the just completed refraction, and if the patient thinks **it is a worthwhile improvement**, then it can be prescribed. (See *Trial Run* on page 68.) If the patient responds that the glasses are better than the refraction, then a change in prescription should not be made, or the refraction should be reworked.

If there is uncertainty about whether the planned change is an improvement for each eye, the comparison between the measured and present prescription can be performed **monocularly**.

When performing either monocular or binocular comparisons, the prescriptions can be shown sequentially using the phoropter alone, or they can be compared by alternating between the phoropter and the current glasses.

If the patient is presbyopic, the patient should similarly be shown the potential change binocularly at near to again make certain it is an improvement.

The refractionist should not feel that anything has been done wrong if the patient states vision is clearer with the current glasses. This can be the case even after a meticulously and beautifully performed refraction.

It is the patient who should decide if the measured change in prescription is made, not the refractionist. The comparison will allow the patient to decide if the improvement in vision will be beneficial, and if it is enough of an improvement to justify the expense.

Note

Showing and comparing lessens the chance the patient will call and say, "I bought these expensive new glasses… and my old glasses are better!"

Trial Run

The purpose of the trial run is to determine if the measured change in prescription will be tolerated by the patient.

In several situations, it is important to **place the planned prescription in a trial frame** and have the patient **take a short walk** before writing the prescription. The planned change may be well tolerated sitting in the exam chair, but walking with the prescription can identify a problem not detectable "in the chair." A change in the astigmatism correction has a greater potential to cause difficulty than a change in the sphere.

The trial run can be presented to the patient as a "**test drive**" and should be done when:

▶ There is a **significant change in the patient's spherical correction**.

▶ There is **more than a small change in cylinder axis or power (especially axis)**.

▶ This is the patient's **first pair of glasses**.

▶ Cylinder is being prescribed for the **first time**.

▶ The patient lost the previous pair of glasses and, therefore, the amount of change cannot be determined.

▶ There is any other concern about the new prescription.

After walking with the new prescription in place, if the patient reports experiencing eyestrain, "pulling," nausea, things looking slanted, an alteration of depth perception ("the floor is coming up to me"), or poorer vision than with the current glasses, you do not want to give that prescription!

When the intended prescription is not tolerated on the trial run, it is very unlikely the patient will adjust to it over time.

If the trial run identifies a problem, the prescription can be **modified** in the trial frame until the patient feels comfortable with it.

Note

It is not helpful to have the patient **sit** with the prescription in the trial frame.

The prescription being tested has already been found to be better in the exam chair. Tolerability is best determined by walking.

The trial run helps greatly to lessen the chance the patient will call and say, "I bought these expensive new glasses… and wearing them makes me dizzy!"

Additional Factors to Consider Prior to Making a Prescription Change

► Does the patient report **any difficulty** functioning with the present glasses?

► **How long** has the patient been wearing the current glasses? The longer a patient has worn a given prescription, the more difficult it may be to adjust to a new one.

► Does the patient need to get new glasses because of **scratches on the lenses** or because he or she would like to get **new frames**? In these situations, there is no need to worry that a change is "too small to make."

► The **magnitude and type** of the measured change. Lesser changes than measured can be made.

► **Cost** considerations must also be taken into account, as purchasing a pair of glasses is not an insignificant expense.

► **The patient**, not the refractionist, should be the one making the final decision about a change in prescription.

New Presbyope

For a **new presbyope**, discuss the pros and cons of the possible methods of correction:

► Over-the-counter reading glasses: Do not hesitate to recommend these if the patient has an insignificant distance correction.

► Using two pairs of glasses: One pair for distance, one pair for near

► Bifocals: Flat-top versus progressive addition lens (PAL)

Note

It is best if you discuss these options with your patient. The type of presbyopic correction can be decided upon with the patient, and the prescription written accordingly.

If an older individual is doing well with a flat-top bifocal, it is best to continue with that type.

Two Myths

When prescribing a patient's **first pair of glasses**, discuss **how often the glasses should be worn** as this will be a concern.

It is often helpful to begin by mentioning two conflicting myths:

1. **Myth 1**: "You should wear the glasses all the time; if you don't, you are straining your eyes."

2. **Myth 2**: "Don't start wearing glasses because your eyes will become weak and dependent on them."

Although well-entrenched in our culture, **neither is correct!**

Glasses, when worn, are simply helping the individual see better. (There are exceptions to this, such as when glasses are being used in the treatment of accommodative esotropia or amblyopia. Another exception is when being used for eye protection.)

The proper instruction, in the usual situation, is that **the glasses should be worn when the individual wants to see more clearly**. This may mean that the glasses are worn all of the time or only for specific tasks such as night driving. Visual need should determine the wearing schedule, **without any concern about hurting or affecting the eyes**.

The "**winter coat analogy**" is one way to clarify this concept for the patient. One knows when a winter coat is needed and, conversely, when it is not.

If one is prescribing glasses for a child or teenager, **it is important to give these instructions to both the child and the parent**.

Special Situations

If a patient has glasses with **prism** that you would like to continue in the new prescription without change, but you are not completely confident in your measurement, write "**duplicate prism**" on the prescription and the optician will be able to do so.

To provide extra **safety, polycarbonate lenses** have traditionally been preferred **for children** and the **monocular patient. Trivex lenses** (PPG Industries) are a newer alternative, having less chromatic aberration than polycarbonate. Fortunately, **standard plastic lenses** also provide a good amount of protection.

Final Considerations

When a change in prescription is being made, it is good to instruct the patient to **purchase only one pair of glasses initially**. If the prescription should need to be modified for whatever reason, only one pair of glasses will then need to be remade. Once the new prescription is successfully worn, the patient can order one or more additional pairs of glasses if desired.

If you are prescribing a PAL for a patient who has never used this type of correction, explain that a **slight tilt up of the chin** (i.e., head tilted slightly back) will usually provide optimal focus for a desktop computer monitor. Some patients do not discover this on their own.

If you are prescribing glasses for a child, **direct your discussion and give the glasses prescription to the child rather than the parent**. The parent will, of course, be listening to every word you say, but the child is your patient and has just cooperated for your exam. Although it will probably not be acknowledged, both the child and the parent will appreciate the consideration and respect inherent in doing so. The child will often immediately give the prescription to the parent, and that is fine.

Instruct the patient to **call you after a few days** if there is any difficulty with the new glasses. The standard optical industry practice is that, if there is a need for a prescription change, the glasses will be remade at no additional cost to the patient within the first month after purchase.

SUBJECTIVE REFRACTION OVER CURRENT LENSES (SPHERICAL OVER-REFRACTION)

▶ Subjective spherical **over-refraction** is performed "over" the patient's current glasses. With the other eye occluded, the patient is shown spherical lenses in front of the glasses lens in the same manner as Step 4 to determine if a change in the spherical part of the correction needs to be made.

▶ Over-refraction can be performed **when a change in the cylinder power and axis is not indicated**. This might be the case if a meticulous refraction was performed 1 year earlier and the patient's acuity is excellent, suggesting that a change in the astigmatism portion of the prescription is not likely to have occurred.

▶ One can use **trial lenses** or lenses mounted on a handle, the latter a "**confirmation test**." For a patient with reasonably good vision, begin by showing a +0.25 and a -0.25 diopter lens to compare. (Begin with +/- 0.50 lenses if vision is somewhat decreased.) If the two choices are of equal clarity, no change in the spherical correction is indicated. If either the choice on the plus side or the minus side is clearer, continue the subjective refraction with lenses on the chosen side.

▶ When over-refracting, try to make sure the patient is looking through the **optical center** of the lens in the glasses.

▶ When testing distance vision over a **PAL**, it is very important to make certain the patient's **chin is not elevated**. If the patient is looking through the intermediate channel, this will prevent determination of the correct distance measurement.

▶ When working with the patient's glasses, one can occlude the eye not being tested with a **hand-held occluder** or a **clip-on occluder**. If the patient holds the occluder, make sure the glasses are in the normal position and are not being pushed closer to the eye. This is especially important with larger prescriptions where a change in **vertex distance** affects the measurement. Also, check to make certain the glasses are not being pushed up so that the patient is looking through the **bifocal** or the **progression in a PAL**. The clip-on occluder does not alter the patient's vertex distance.

▶ Over-refraction can be used to evaluate the **reading prescription** as well as the distance prescription.

▶ When over-refracting for near vision with reading glasses, make sure the glasses are **positioned where they are usually worn**. A change in position alters the effective power of the lenses.

▶ Over-refraction can also be used when measuring for **computer glasses**. One technique is to **place the near card on the slit lamp chin rest**, with the position of the slit lamp adjusted to simulate the distance and height of the patient's desktop computer monitor.

Note

As a screening method to determine if previously undetected astigmatism might be present, a +0.50 diopter cylindrical lens can be held up, at varying axes, **over a spherical correction**.

NEAR VISION

▶ The **Jaeger** (pronounced "Yaager") **system of notation** (e.g., J1+, J2, J10) is used for near to readily differentiate it from distance acuity.

▶ When determining the proper correction needed for reading, **ask patients to hold the near card at their ideal reading distance**. Clarify that you are not asking that the card be held the distance where things seem most clear with the current glasses. The ideal reading distance is used (rather than the 14 inches specified on some near cards) because that is where most reading will occur. (It is, however, at 14 inches that the Snellen equivalent designations are valid.)

▶ When testing near vision, it is usually best to measure **each eye** individually. This is helpful even though the prescribed Add will almost always be the same for each eye.

▶ If an asymmetric Add is measured, this suggests that the **distance prescription** (that it is being added to) may be incorrect.

▶ The goal of near refraction is to find the correction that makes the numbers or letters on the near card **clearer, not larger**. The correction for near is simply supplementing or replacing the individual's diminished accommodative ability—an ability which, when it was functioning fully, focused but did not enlarge small print.

▶ An Add that **magnifies** is overly strong. This is not desirable because, as the Add increases, the **closer and narrower** the reading range becomes.

▶ Before prescribing an Add or reading glasses, it is very helpful to evaluate the **range of clear near vision** with the planned correction. The range is determined by asking the patient to bring the near card forward, stopping when the numbers or letters blur. The patient is then asked to push the card away, stopping when blurring occurs. The reading range is optimal when the patient's ideal reading position is halfway between these near and far positions. (See *Presbyopia* on page 14.)

USING THE TRIAL FRAME

▶ Adjust the trial frame so it is **sitting properly** on the patient's face with the lenses centered on each pupil.

▶ Place the **spherical correction** in the clip at the back of the trial frame and place the **cylinder** in the clip at the front of the trial frame so the axis can be adjusted.

▶ Keep the trial lenses organized in the trial lens drawer by **placing each lens in its correct slot immediately after use**.

▶ Keep the trial lenses **clean**.

Refraction Reminders

- As with the medical problems that present to us, refraction and prescribing glasses involve **history, examination, diagnosis, and treatment decisions**.
- The process is not only measurement, but **problem solving**.
- Often, the diagnosis of the patient's problem can be made from the **history**.
- The goal is to give the **simplest system that satisfies that individual patient's visual needs**.
- **Show, compare, and discuss with the patient** any change you are considering.
- **An optimal glasses prescription is of maximal importance to our patients.**
- **With a well-performed refraction, we are helping our patients see more clearly—without medicines or surgery.**
- **Our patients benefit from a correct glasses prescription all day, every day.**
- **The art of refraction is mastered by practice!**

CHAPTER 3

Case Studies

The case studies are presented in a **question-and-answer** format. They are **composite cases** representing situations that will present to the refractionist. **The principles discussed apply equally to the plus and minus cylinder methods.**

Kolker RJ, Kolker AF. *Subjective Refraction and Prescribing Glasses: The Number One (or Number Two) Guide to Practical Techniques and Principles (pp 75–119).*
© 2018 Taylor & Francis Group.

Myopia

Myopia Case 1

A 24-year-old male myope, despite seeing reasonably well at distance without correction, is **"soaking up" minus spherical power during subjective refraction**. Why is this happening, and what can be done to determine if it is needed?

· · · · · ·
Answer

It is important, when performing subjective refraction, to be concerned about giving the patient too much minus spherical correction. **Over-minusing** occurs as a result of the patient accommodating during the refraction. This is especially a concern with a younger patient because a young person has a great deal of accommodative ability. There is a tendency for the extra minus power to be preferred by the patient because the letters on the acuity chart will look smaller and darker and, thus, "better."

There are several techniques that can be employed to try to prevent over-minusing during subjective refraction:

▶ The patient should be instructed, and reminded, to compare only the clarity of the choices being shown. It should be emphasized that if a given choice only makes the letters **smaller and darker**, it should be considered "the same."

▶ The refractionist should make certain the additional minus is resulting in improved ability to read the **acuity chart**.

▶ **Fogging** techniques can be employed so that the patient is moving from a position of extra plus. (See *Over-Minusing* on page 60.)

▶ The red-green **duochrome test** can be used. (See *Over-Minusing* on page 60.)

▶ A **cycloplegic refraction** can be performed. (See *The Three Types of Refraction* on page 32.)

Myopia Case 2

A 75-year-old female is found to have a -1.00 diopter change in refractive error in each eye from the prescription of 1 year ago. What are the possible etiologies of this **myopic shift**? What are the considerations before giving her a prescription for a new pair of glasses incorporating this myopic shift?

• • • • • •
Answer

Possible etiologies include a nuclear sclerotic **cataract**, the onset or worsening of control of **diabetes mellitus**, a recent **scleral buckle**, some **medications** (e.g., **tetracycline**, **topiramate**), and **hyperbaric oxygen** treatment.

If it is determined that the myopic shift is due to a **cataract**, it should be explained to her that the change in prescription will offset, but not overcome, the cataract (unless it is very mild).

The change in prescription measured should be shown to her binocularly at distance and near. A decision will have to be made, with the patient, whether the change will allow satisfactory performance of activities of daily living.

If, after discussion, it is unclear whether the vision will or will not be satisfactory with the new prescription, it is sometimes best to make the change. That way, both you and the patient will know that if there is continued difficulty while wearing the new prescription, cataract surgery is indeed indicated.

If it is determined the myopic shift has resulted from **diabetes**, it is usually best to remeasure once the glucose level is stabilized.

If a **systemic medication** is considered to be the etiology of the myopic shift, a decision about changing the glasses will depend upon the length of time the patient is expected to be on the medication. Discussion with the prescribing doctor is at times very helpful.

Myopia Case 3

A 48-year-old male myope, without separate reading glasses or a bifocal, is having no trouble reading. Why? (He is certainly at the age one would expect him to have symptomatic presbyopia.)

• • • • • •
Answer

If he is wearing glasses for myopia, almost certainly his **myopic refractive error is not fully corrected**. He can read at near because of the myopia that remains uncorrected.

In this situation, if the patient feels he is seeing satisfactorily at distance and near, it is often best to not give the additional minus to fully correct the distance refractive error. **Keeping him "under-minused"** allows him to defer moving to a bifocal or progressive addition lens (PAL) for a little while. If he were to be given the full myopic prescription, almost certainly a bifocal or PAL would be needed.

If he is not functioning satisfactorily at distance, then the full myopic prescription can be given, with the addition of a bifocal or PAL. The decision about when to no longer use a single-vision lens is best made with the patient.

Note

An extension of this concept can be seen in individuals with myopia who take off their glasses to read. They are reading with what can be termed their "**natural nearsightedness**."

Myopia Case 4

A 37-year-old female myope seeing well at distance with her glasses is having trouble reading. Is this presbyopia?

. . . . . .
Answer

For someone 37 years of age, presbyopia is not the most likely diagnosis. It is much more likely she is **over-minused** at distance. Her trouble reading is, most probably, the result of having to use her accommodative ability to offset the excessive minus in her glasses. She, therefore, does not have enough accommodation left to use for reading.

> ### Note
>
> Let the patient know that the new glasses you will be prescribing, with less minus sphere, may require a little adjustment period for seeing clearly at distance, as **accommodative tone** may take a little time to relax.

Myopia Case 5

A 55-year-old male with high myopia presents for routine examination. You determine that he does not need a change in glasses and that his eyes are in excellent health. When discussing those results, **what else should you tell him**?

. . . . . .
Answer

Because an individual with **high myopia** has an increased risk of a retinal tear and subsequent detachment, it is important to instruct him to call immediately should he have the **onset of new floaters, flashes, or a change in side vision**. This reminder should be repeated and reinforced when you see him in the future.

Myopia Case 6

A 30-year-old female who has never worn glasses is examined and found to have a **small amount of myopia**. She says she does not feel she needs distance glasses. Should you prescribe them?

• • • • • •
Answer

If she feels she is seeing satisfactorily at distance and you have found only a small myopic correction, it is fine for her to continue to function **without distance glasses**.

Were you to prescribe the glasses for her, the proper instructions would be that they do not need to be worn all the time—only when she wanted their help. She has indicated it is unlikely she would use them, so it would probably be an unnecessary expense.

Myopia Case 7

A 35-year-old male wearing glasses for myopia is examined, and you measure a **very slight increase in his myopic correction. Should you make it?**

• • • • • •
Answer

The best way to determine if this change should be made is to **show** it to him and **let him decide** whether he feels it is a significant enough improvement to warrant the purchase of a new pair of glasses.

Note

This is a good rule-of-thumb to follow for any anticipated change in prescription.

Hyperopia

Hyperopia Case 1

A 37-year-old male with a new, single-vision, hyperopic correction in his glasses is seeing well at distance, but is having difficulty reading. Is this presbyopia?

• • • • • •
Answer

He most likely has hyperopia that is not being fully corrected by his glasses. He is, therefore, using his accommodative ability to correct the **latent hyperopia**, leaving an insufficient amount of accommodation for reading.

When measuring to uncover latent hyperopia, one may perform a **cycloplegic refraction** or "**push plus.**" The latter is accomplished during a noncycloplegic refraction by giving as much plus spherical power as the patient will tolerate without causing blurring or discomfort. (See *Hyperopia Case 3* on page 82.)

Note

Latent hyperopia can (not uncommonly) be present in individuals who see well at distance without glasses and are not known to be hyperopic.

Hyperopia Case 2

A **50-year-old female** who has never needed distance glasses and is successfully using over-the-counter (OTC) reading glasses is **now beginning to have trouble with distance vision**. Why, and what might you recommend?

• • • • • •
Answer

Her difficulty at distance is almost certainly due to **latent hyperopia that has now become manifest**. Prior to age 50 years, she was able to use her accommodative ability to correct her distance vision, but now there is not enough accommodation left to do so.

If she does not want a bifocal or PAL and does not mind having two pairs of glasses, there is an inexpensive way to correct her vision for distance and near. If she has a low and symmetrical amount of hyperopia, with no astigmatism, she can use OTC reading glasses for distance. For example, she may do well using a +1.00 pair for distance and a +3.00 pair for near.

Hyperopia Case 3

A 25-year-old male found to have **latent hyperopia** was recently given a glasses prescription following a **cycloplegic refraction**. He is now complaining that he **cannot tolerate the new glasses**. What should be done?

• • • • • •
Answer

He should return for a **post-cycloplegic refraction**.

If a significant amount of plus sphere, not previously worn, is found on a cycloplegic refraction, it is best to bring the patient back for a post-cycloplegic refraction before writing the final prescription. The purpose is to determine how much of the full cycloplegic refraction can be tolerated.

A lesser amount than the full hyperopic correction may need to be prescribed initially because the long-standing **accommodative tone**, which has been used to self-correct the latent hyperopia, can be resistant to relaxation. Over time, this tone will decrease and, subsequently, additional plus can be added in stages until the full hyperopic correction is accepted. (See *Hyperopia Case 1* on page 81.)

Hyperopia Case 4

A 64-year-old female returns for her annual visit and is found to have developed a **hyperopic shift** in her prescription. What are two possible etiologies?

• • • • • •
Answer

1. Macular edema
2. Recent initiation of treatment, or treatment change, for diabetes mellitus that had previously caused a myopic shift (now reversed).

Hyperopia Case 5

A 6-year-old female is examined and found to have a refractive error of +1.25 in each eye. **Should glasses be given?**

. . . . . .
Answer

Because of her young age, and if strabismus is not a factor, glasses **should not** be given for this refractive error. She has ample accommodation to correct the hyperopia, and it will be invoked without any conscious effort.

Note

It is also not necessary to give a correction for a **small amount of astigmatism** at this age.

Astigmatism

Astigmatism Case 1

A 35-year-old male patient calls, having just begun wearing the new glasses you prescribed.

His previous prescription: OD -2.25 + 1.00 × 90°

OS -2.00 + 1.00 × 90°

The prescription you gave: OD -2.50 + 1.75 × 75°

OS -1.75 + 1.50 × 105°

He says that, with the new glasses, **the top of his desk looks slanted and, when walking, he has some nausea and the floor seems to be rising**.

What is the most likely cause of his symptoms?

Answer

The symptoms are almost certainly due to the change made in the **astigmatism correction** in the new prescription.

The astigmatic portion of a glasses prescription is the most prone to cause difficulty. A change in cylinder axis, especially with higher cylinder powers, is always a concern. A "**trial run**" prior to prescribing may very well have avoided his problems. (See *Trial Run* on page 68.)

Astigmatism Case 2

A 26-year-old female who has never worn glasses presents complaining of decreased distance vision. If retinoscopy is not performed, and an autorefractor is not available, **how do you determine if cylinder is present**?

Answer

(See *Sixteen Tips for Accurate Subjective Refraction Results, Tip 9* on page 64.)

Astigmatism Case 3

A 34-year-old female, at the phoropter, is beginning subjective refraction with the following prescription in one of her eyes: -3.50 + 0.50 × 180°.

The spherical correction in Step 1 is determined to be -3.00, and in Step 2, the axis remains unchanged. (See *The Four Steps of Subjective Refraction* on page 33.)

You begin modifying the cylinder power of +0.50 × 180 with the Jackson cross cylinder, and she says the choice with the red dot is clearer. Therefore, you lessen the cylinder power to +0.25 × 180°.

On the next series, she again chooses the red dot and you lessen the cylinder power to 0.00 × 180°, and add +0.25 power to the sphere.

On the next sequence of choices she once again chooses the red dot, but **you are working with plus cylinders and cannot go any lower. What can you do?**

· · · · · ·
Answer

The patient is choosing less plus cylinder power when the cylinder power is already at 0 and therefore cannot go any lower. This dilemma is resolved by understanding that the patient is actually choosing plus cylinder power 90 degrees away. In this case, change the axis from 180 degrees to 90 degrees, dial in +0.50 diopter of cylinder power at 90 degrees, adjust the sphere by 0.25 diopter, and then begin again to refine cylinder axis and power. (See *The Rule* below.)

Note

The Rule: **If a patient chooses "less than 0" cylinder power**, the axis should be shifted 90 degrees from its current location. This applies to both the plus and minus cylinder methods. (See *Sixteen Tips for Accurate Subjective Refraction Results, Tip 9* on page 64.)

Astigmatism Case 4

A 25-year-old female myope, who previously had a small amount of astigmatism, is **choosing a large amount of plus cylinder power during subjective refraction**. Why?

Answer

It may be that there has simply been an increase in the astigmatism, or a corneal problem such as keratoconus could be the cause. However, it is important to make sure this is not the result of **over-minusing the sphere**, which will necessitate an increase in cylinder power.

For every 0.50 diopter a patient with plus cylinder is over-minused, the cylinder power needs to be increased by 1 diopter to maintain the spherical equivalent and keep the circle of least confusion on the retina. (See *Spherical Equivalent of an Astigmatic Prescription* on page 23.)

For example, if a patient has a true refractive error of -3.50 **+0.50** × 180°, the spherical equivalent of the correct prescription is -3.25.

If the sphere is over-minused by -0.50 diopter (to -4.00), the patient will choose an increase in cylinder power of +1.00 diopter (to +1.50), with a resulting spherical equivalent of -3.25.

The increased cylinder power will be preferred because letters will appear most clear at the spherical equivalent.

This results in a measured correction of -4.00 **+1.50** × 180°.

In summary, over-minusing the sphere results in an incorrect measurement of cylinder power.

Note

Conversely, if sphere is over-minused in the **minus cylinder method**, the patient will choose less than the true cylinder power. (See *Over-Minusing* on page 60.)

Astigmatism Case 5

A 45-year-old, newly presbyopic male is examined and found to have, in each eye, a distance refractive correction of plano +0.50 × 90° and a near correction of +1.50 +0.50 × 90°. He has never had distance glasses and his only difficulty is with reading. **What should you give?**

· · · · · ·
Answer

If he feels he is seeing fine at distance and would simply like help with reading, he may do quite well with **OTC reading glasses**. A strength of +1.75 would be recommended based on the spherical equivalent of the near measurement. It is not necessary to give a prescription incorporating the astigmatism correction unless his reading or distance acuity is significantly improved with the addition of the cylinder, and he wants it.

Astigmatism Case 6

A 14-year-old female, who has not had a previous refraction, complains of trouble seeing at distance. Subjective refraction results in the following prescription:

OD -1.75 + 0.50 × 100°   VA 20/20

OS -1.50 sphere   VA 20/25 (pinhole 20/20)

No organic etiology is found to explain the lesser acuity in the left eye.

What should be the next step?

· · · · · ·
Answer

Because the astigmatic correction for a patient is **often symmetrical**, a helpful next step would be to look for that possibility. Complete symmetry would indicate a refractive error for the left eye of -1.75 + 0.50 × 80°. **When symmetrical, the axes add to 180 degrees.** Repeat subjective refraction for the left eye could begin with that prescription, and note that the correction originally found is the spherical equivalent of the new starting point.

Presbyopia

Presbyopia Case 1

A 45-year-old female presents with the complaint when trying to read, "**My arms aren't long enough.**"

What is the diagnosis and what should you prescribe?

• • • • • •
Answer

Her symptom is the result of **presbyopia**.

The patient's age is **45 years**. This is usually when the initial correction of presbyopia is necessary, not age 40 years as is often stated. If presbyopic symptoms occur before age 45 years, make certain the patient is not over-minused or a latent hyperope. These may be the cause of the earlier-than-usual onset of presbyopic symptoms. Conversely, if a patient is reading satisfactorily without correction in the late 40s, it is very likely some uncorrected myopia is present.

The treatment for presbyopia would seem to be very simple, but surprisingly there are **four categories of solutions, and additional choices within the categories**.

The **four categories** are as follows:

1. **Give nothing**: If she has mild-to-moderate myopia and **has been taking her distance glasses off for reading**, it is fine to have her continue to do so. When the glasses are off, she is reading with her "**natural nearsightedness.**"

2. **Give reading glasses**: She can be given a **prescription for reading glasses** or, if appropriate, instructed to purchase **OTC** reading glasses.

   Three things to consider with regard to OTC reading glasses:

   a. OTC reading glasses are sometimes referred to as **drugstore reading glasses, readers, cheaters**, or **magnifiers**. Although OTC reading glasses are called **magnifiers**, their purpose is **not magnification**. Their function is to **supplement** the patient's diminished focusing ability. That focusing ability, before it was lost, focused the print but did not enlarge it.

   The proper strength for OTC reading glasses is determined by finding the **amount of plus power that best focuses the reading material without magnifying it**. The reason to refrain from giving additional plus power, which would produce magnification, is that it would result in an **unnecessarily closer and narrower reading range**. An exception to this is for a patient with low vision where magnification is purposefully given.

b. OTC reading glasses are appropriate when **three criteria** are met:

- ◆ The patient must be essentially **emmetropic at distance**. (If glasses are worn to correct a distance refractive error, an Add is typically prescribed.)

- ◆ The two eyes must be reasonably **symmetrical** in their refractive status. OTC reading glasses have the same strength lens for each eye.

- ◆ The patient must have **no astigmatism**, or an insignificant amount. OTC reading glasses have spherical plus power only.

Note

When these **three criteria** are met, OTC reading glasses can be recommended with confidence. The strength designation found on the glasses can be relied upon, the quality of the lenses is good, and there is a significant cost saving for the patient.

c. **Three types of OTC reading glasses** are made, and it is helpful to discuss with the patient the pros and cons of each type to determine which is likely to work best:

- ◆ **Half-glasses**:

   Pro: Allows for distance viewing over the top of the glasses.

   Con: Some individuals prefer to not have this style.

- ◆ **Full reading glasses**:

   Pro: Gives the patient a larger reading area than the half-glasses.

   Con: The glasses need to be removed for distance viewing.

- ◆ **Plano bifocals** (plano at top; flat-top bifocal at bottom):

   Pro: Allows the patient to alternate between distance and near.

   Con: Some patients prefer to not have bifocals.

Note

It is helpful to write down for the patient the **strength and type** of reading glasses decided upon. When doing so, it is best to write "**OTC**" clearly on the prescription to avoid confusion if it is taken to an optical shop.

3. **Give two pairs of glasses, one for distance and one for near**: This choice may be especially appropriate if distance glasses are used only for certain tasks, such as driving. The patient may then prefer to have separate distance and reading glasses, using each pair when appropriate.

   This choice is probably not best if someone, at work or home, has a need to frequently alternate vision from distance to near and vice versa. This would necessitate an inconvenient amount of switching between the two pairs.

   Two pairs of glasses may also be preferred by a patient who is overly concerned about using a bifocal. A new presbyope may sometimes choose to begin with separate reading glasses for this reason, knowing a change to a bifocal or PAL can be made if switching back and forth between the two pairs of glasses is occurring too often.

4. **Give bifocal or multifocal glasses**: This choice works best for most people as it is the simplest and most efficient way for the presbyope to have **best corrected vision both at distance and near**. In daily life, we are constantly alternating our gaze from far to near, as well as in-between. Teachers are a prime example because they often have to read and look out at a classroom of students in the same setting. Also, some individuals like to sit and simultaneously read or knit while watching TV.

   It is good to be aware that, for some patients, the initial prescription of a bifocal is a cause for **worry or even mild distress**. Some are concerned about adjusting to them, while others consider it an unpleasant indication that they are getting older. If these concerns are detected, gentle reassurance can be quite helpful.

   It is important to discuss with the patient that there are three primary ways a presbyopic Add can be given. It can be given as a **standard bifocal, a trifocal, or a PAL**, the latter sometimes referred to as a **no-line bifocal**. It is best to discuss the pros and cons of each of these options with the patient to determine which is most appropriate.

   The **standard bifocal** has a line and may be given as a **flat-top segment** or, less often, as an **executive bifocal**. In the latter, the bifocal segment occupies the entire lower portion of the lens. The intermediate distance is not corrected by a standard bifocal.

   The **trifocal** has three distinct segments, with two separating lines. The third (middle) lens corrects the **intermediate distance**. Gaps between distance and intermediate, as well as between intermediate and near, do exist. The trifocal is prescribed with much less frequency now that the PAL is available.

The **PAL** is a **graduated multifocal**. Plus power increases progressively from the distance portion at the top of the lens to the full strength Add at the bottom. This lens allows one to focus from distance to near, without any gaps, by looking further down the lens.

Note

It is important to let the patient known that, when a progressive lens is working properly, **distance vision** should be clear when he or she is looking straight ahead, **near vision** should be clear when he or she is looking down in the usual reading position, and it is only in the **intermediate area** where some adjustment with chin-up positioning needs to be made. The closer the object, the higher the chin needs to be. After a short while, positioning for the intermediate distance should happen essentially automatically.

The great advantage of the PAL is that it allows clear vision at all distances, allowing one to **function very similarly to how one did prior to the onset of presbyopia**!

It needs to be mentioned to the patient that there is an **inherent blur at the sides** with the PAL. This does necessitate straight-ahead viewing for most things, especially reading. Most patients are able to adjust to this easily as now movement of the head is necessary as one reads across a page rather than moving only one's eyes. Of note, the **free-form progressive lens** has greatly improved side vision in the PAL.

Note

Bifocal and multifocal glasses do not usually work well for patients who watch TV while lying in bed. These patients will have difficulty seeing the TV screen clearly because, when in the supine position, they are looking through the Add rather than the distance portion of the lens.

In summary, it is very important to determine, **with the patient**, which of these options will most effectively maximize daily visual functioning. (See *Presbyopia* on page 14.)

Presbyopia Case 2

A 45-year-old male for whom you have just recommended OTC reading glasses asks, **"Will using reading glasses weaken my eyes?"**

. . . . . .
Answer

No, it will not. There will be a normal decrease in accommodative ability over time, and this will occur at the same rate whether reading glasses are used or not. It is expected that, in the future, the patient will become more dependent on reading glasses. This is simply the result of presbyopia's normal progression.

> ### *Note*
>
> An occasional patient will report that, despite difficulty reading, recommended reading glasses are not being used because of the mistaken belief that this will "keep my eyes strong."

Presbyopia Case 3

A 50-year-old female who received reading glasses several years prior complains that she **now needs her reading glasses to see food clearly when eating**. Why is this happening?

. . . . . .
Answer

The patient can be reassured that what she is experiencing is normal. In a sense, reading glasses are misnamed; they should be called **"near glasses."** They are simply making up for the accommodative ability that has been lost, and that accommodative ability was used to bring anything at near into focus, including food.

Presbyopia Case 4

A 50-year-old male presbyope is examined, and it is found that he needs an increase in the strength of his OTC reading glasses. He asks, "**Can I still use my old reading glasses that are less strong, or will that hurt my eyes?**"

• • • • • •
Answer

He **can** continue to use the older reading glasses as long as he finds that the glasses are providing satisfactory vision for reading and not causing eyestrain. He is not doing any harm by using them.

Presbyopia Case 5

A **55-year-old female with moderately high myopia** is successfully using PALs for normal reading. She complains she is having **difficulty threading a needle**. What might you recommend?

• • • • • •
Answer

The simplest solution is to recommend that she **take off her glasses** for threading a needle. In doing so, she is using her "**natural nearsightedness**" to see up close and no accommodation or supplemental plus power is needed. The needle and thread will need to be held closer than the normal reading distance.

This strategy will also be beneficial when she is trying to read **very small print**, or when it is necessary to read something **positioned** so high the Add cannot be used.

Presbyopia Case 6

A 45-year-old emmetropic male presents with three complaints:

1. "I am having trouble reading the menu in a dimly lit restaurant."

2. "I have some difficulty reading early in the morning and late at night."

3. "I cannot see clearly when reading in bed at night."

What is the diagnosis and how should he be managed?

 • • • • • •
Answer

These are common symptoms of diminished accommodative ability at the **onset of presbyopia**. They occur because (in response to each question):

1. **In dim illumination**, the pupils will dilate, resulting in a loss of the **pinhole effect of miosis**. (With diminished accommodative ability, the pinhole effect aids the ability to read clearly.)

Note

The corollary: **In bright light**, reading is often easier for a presbyope.

2. Accommodation tends to function as we often do. There can be a little **sluggishness** in the morning and **fatigue** late at night!

3. When reading in bed at night, one tends to hold the reading material **closer** than when sitting up during the day. Closer requires more accommodation.

For this patient, an emmetrope at age 45 years, usually a pair of +1.50 OTC reading glasses will work quite well. (See *Four Points About Correcting Presbyopia With an Add* on page 16.)

Presbyopia Case 7

A 44-year-old emmetropic female complains that it **takes a few seconds for her vision to become clear when looking across the room after reading**. What is the etiology, and should glasses be given for this?

. . . . . .
Answer

Her symptom is due to **early presbyopia**. Her remaining accommodation is working very hard to allow her to read and, because of this extra effort, it takes a few seconds for it to relax when she looks up.

If this symptom is something she has simply noticed but is not causing any inconvenience or difficulty, reading glasses can be **deferred**. However, if she has also noticed some difficulty with small print or would like to eliminate this problem, then OTC reading glasses can be **recommended**.

Presbyopia Case 8

A 50-year-old male emmetropic presbyope using OTC reading glasses asks, "**Why was I able to read without my reading glasses when I was at the beach?**" Why was he able to do so?

. . . . . .
Answer

He was experiencing the **pinhole effect**, without using the pinhole occluder! In bright sunlight, the pupil reaches a level of miosis that produces the pinhole effect. Through a pinhole, only the central rays from an object being viewed are able to enter the eye. These central rays, unlike more peripheral ones, do not require refraction.

Note
Squinting is another method of producing the pinhole effect.

Presbyopia Case 9

A 50-year-old female emmetropic presbyope using +1.50 OTC reading glasses has noticed that moving the glasses farther down her nose improves clarity. Why, and what should be recommended?

· · · · · ·
Answer

Her clarity is improved because the longer vertex distance (the distance between the cornea and the lens) is optically adding plus power. Her history is indicating she needs stronger reading glasses. An improvement in clarity, with the glasses at their usual position, will be achieved by increasing the strength to +2.00.

Presbyopia Correction

Presbyopia Correction Case 1

A 60-year-old male using a **flat-top bifocal** is having **difficulty reading** with the recent prescription you gave him. His distance vision is fine. What should you do?

Answer

Additional information is needed, and will likely indicate where the problem lies. Three potential problems can be considered:

1. He should be asked whether clarity is improved by **pushing the reading material farther away** (indicating a bifocal that is too weak) or **bringing it closer** (indicating a bifocal that is too strong).

2. The line for the flat-top bifocal segment should typically be **positioned at the lower lid margin**. If it appears on your examination that the segment is too low, he should be asked whether he has noticed that pushing the glasses up or tilting his chin up has helped him read more easily.

Note

Because glasses have a tendency to slide down the nose in some individuals, the **working position** of the bifocal may be lower than intended.

3. It is also important to check that the **bottom portion of the lenses are angled inwardly**. This inward slant is called the **pantoscopic tilt**. The lack of a proper pantoscopic tilt can make reading more difficult, and correcting it can significantly enhance the ability to read comfortably.

Note

Always remember that a bifocal **Add** is literally **added to the distance prescription. If the distance prescription is incorrect, the reading portion of the bifocal will be incorrect.**

Presbyopia Correction Case 2

A 70-year-old presbyopic female whom you have **changed from a flat-top bifocal to a PAL** is not doing well. How should her problem be approached?

Answer

The first consideration is whether she should have been changed from a standard bifocal to a PAL. In general, if a patient is doing perfectly well and has no complaints in a standard bifocal, it may be best to continue with that type. However, if there is a need to correct the intermediate distance (e.g., for computer work), it is very reasonable to make the change.

It is important to determine the nature of her difficulty with the new prescription:

- ▶ Is she bothered by the inherent **blur at the sides** of a PAL?
- ▶ Does she need to assume an abnormal **head position** for distance viewing or when reading?
- ▶ Is there a proper **pantoscopic tilt**?
- ▶ How long has she had the new glasses? There is an **adjustment period** for a progressive bifocal, which can be up to 2 weeks in some individuals.
- ▶ Finally, the new lenses should be measured in the lensometer to be certain the prescription was **filled correctly.**

If the problem cannot be identified or if it is determined that a patient cannot tolerate a PAL, it is best to change back to a standard bifocal. The optician will typically remake the glasses with a flat-top bifocal **without an additional charge**. However, the patient will have paid a premium price for the PAL.

Presbyopia Correction Case 3

A 55-year-old female flat-top bifocal wearer is having difficulty at a desktop computer. What are some possible solutions?

Answer

The monitor for a desktop computer is usually located beyond the normal reading distance. This area is referred to as the **intermediate distance** and is not able to be viewed clearly with either the top (for distance) or bottom (for near) portion of the standard bifocal.

There are three possible solutions for her:

1. A **trifocal** can be prescribed. The middle segment will allow the intermediate distance to be viewed clearly.

2. The **most-often** used solution is to change to a PAL. The patient needs to be instructed to elevate her chin slightly so that she is viewing the monitor through the graduated portion of the lens.

Note

If she has a problem with her neck so that the **chin-up position** poses a difficulty, neither the trifocal nor the PAL will be the best choice.

3. If she does not want either of these two options, a separate pair of "**computer glasses**" can be prescribed for her. Computer glasses have the **intermediate correction at the top of the lens** and the reading correction at the bottom. The computer monitor will be seen clearly **when looking straight ahead**, without the necessity of elevating her chin.

Four notes about prescribing computer glasses:

1. It is often **best to not give a single-vision prescription** that only corrects the intermediate distance. Although the intermediate prescription will function well for the computer screen, if the patient should print some material, it is not easily read in the absence of a near correction.

2. It is often best to give computer glasses as a **PAL or standard bifocal**. A progressive bifocal has the advantage of having no gaps from the computer screen to the reading distance.

3. If the computer glasses prescription contains an Add, it will be an **odd-looking Add**. It will typically be **one-half of the patient's normal Add**. This is because one-half of the full Add has been incorporated into the top part of the prescription, leaving the other half to be added to it at the bottom.

4. A helpful technique to help decide how strong to make the top portion of the computer glasses (for the intermediate distance) is to use a near card propped on the chin rest of the slit lamp. The slit lamp can be positioned to simulate the distance and height of the patient's computer monitor. With this simulation, a measurement of the optimal intermediate correction can be made. (See *Computer Glasses* on page 22.)

Presbyopia Correction Case 4

A **45-year-old emmetropic female** using +1.50 OTC reading glasses very successfully for reading complains that she is having **difficulty threading a needle**. What are the possible solutions?

Answer

Three possible solutions:

1. Have her purchase a separate pair of stronger OTC reading glasses.
2. Have her thread the needle with the current reading glasses under a very strong light.
3. If the need to thread a needle is a very occasional occurrence and she has several pairs of +1.50 readers at home, a creative solution is to use two pairs of reading glasses at the same time. Some patients make this discovery on their own!

Presbyopia Correction Case 5

A 60-year-old priest, when preaching, is having **difficulty reading his sermons** while wearing his flat-top bifocal. What should you do?

Answer

The most likely cause of his difficulty is that the podium he is using is positioned at the intermediate distance, beyond the normal near reading distance. Two possible solutions are as follows:

1. Change to a **PAL** (or a trifocal) so that the intermediate distance can be viewed clearly.
2. If he prefers, a separate pair of "sermon glasses" can be given. This pair will have the full distance correction at the top so the congregation can be seen clearly. **The Add will be half the strength of the Add in his regular glasses** so he will be able to read his sermon notes on the podium.

Note

These same strategies can be beneficial for a **musician** whose music stand is positioned at the intermediate distance.

Presbyopia Correction Case 6

A 50-year-old male musician who plays the **French horn** is having difficulty seeing the **sheet music that is positioned on top of the instrument**. He is currently wearing a flat-top bifocal. How might you help him?

. . . . . .
Answer

When a bifocal Add is incorporated into a lens, it is placed at the bottom portion of the lens because that is the position through which reading material is usually viewed. However, for special needs, the **location of the bifocal** can be changed.

The French horn player would benefit by having the **bifocal at the top portion of the lenses**. In past years, **meter readers** often required this location for a bifocal. Special glasses such as these are termed **occupational bifocals**. Additionally, in the same pair of glasses, the French horn player and the meter reader can continue to have a bifocal at the bottom of the lenses as well!

An **atypical bifocal location** can also be helpful for those individuals who play **golf**. A bifocal positioned in one corner of the lens will not interfere with seeing the golf ball when looking down, but it will allow viewing of the scorecard when looking to the side.

Presbyopia Correction Case 7

Which is more likely to cause a problem for a patient, a bifocal that is **too weak or one that is too strong**?

. . . . . .
Answer

An **overly strong bifocal** is more likely to be bothersome to a patient than a bifocal that is too weak. A closer and narrower reading range (a stronger bifocal) is typically tolerated less well than a farther and wider range (a weaker bifocal).

Also, OTC reading glasses that are being used successfully **for both reading and desktop computing** may not function as well for the computer if they are strengthened because the reading range will become closer and narrower.

Presbyopia Correction Case 8

A 45-year-old male, who is a new bifocal wearer, reports that his bifocals are working very well for most of his activities. However, he has found that his vision is not clear in two situations: **viewing the stage from his theater balcony seat** and **watching TV while lying in bed at night**. What is the most likely cause of his difficulties? What are possible solutions?

Answer

In both situations, the blurring is the result of **gaze being directed through the bottom portion of the lens**—the area designed for near vision.

Two techniques, neither an ideal solution, can be used to redirect his gaze through the top portion of the lens. He can adopt a chin-down position or, alternatively, move the glasses further down on his nose. For prolonged viewing, both may be uncomfortable, and moving the glasses lower on the nose increases the vertex distance, itself a cause of blurring with stronger prescriptions.

If he will be engaging in these activities with some frequency, it would be best to prescribe an additional **distance-only pair of glasses**.

Refraction

Refraction Case 1

A 68-year-old patient gives **frustratingly inconsistent responses during subjective refraction**. What should you do?

. . . . . .
Answer

(See *Sixteen Tips for Accurate Subjective Refraction Results, Tip 10* on page 64.)

Refraction Case 2

A 55-year-old female, for whom you performed a meticulous refraction 2 weeks ago, calls on the phone and says, "**The new glasses you gave me are not good. I can't see well with them.**" What should you do?

. . . . . .
Answer

First, **obtain a good history**:

► Is her difficulty at distance, at near, or both?

► Has she checked to see whether the problem is in one eye or both?

► What are the symptoms she is experiencing: eye strain, objects slanting, nausea, etc?

► How long has she had the new pair?

► Where were the glasses made?

It is almost always necessary to have the patient **return to the office** to be re-evaluated:

► Ask her to **bring both the old and the new glasses, and measure both.**

► If she states that her old glasses are better than the new, **measure her acuity with each pair in the office**. Occasionally, you (and the patient) will find that the new glasses are indeed clearer at distance and near, and only some **reassurance** was needed.

► A **repeat refraction** is usually necessary.

► If you identify the problem and determine that the glasses need to be remade, there will traditionally be **no additional charge to the patient by the optician** if it is within the first 30 days after purchase.

Note

Some opticians allow a longer period of time, and others may extend the 30-day limit depending on individual circumstances.

It is also customary for there to be no charge by the prescriber for this type of return visit.

If you find that the optician has made an error, which is quite rare, it is important to handle this **kindly** and **respectfully**.

If you are **unable to identify the problem** after re-refraction, it is often best to **default back to the old glasses prescription**. This is especially good to do if the complaint is, "My old glasses are better than the new ones." (See *Show and Compare What You Plan to Give—Always!* on page 66.)

Refraction Case 3

A 36-year-old female returns 1 year after an excellent refraction by you with the complaint of recently noting slight difficulty with distance vision. What **type of refraction might you do** this year?

• • • • • •
Answer

It may not be necessary to change the cylinder power and axis determined 1 year earlier. The refraction can begin with a spherical **over-refraction**. (See *Subjective Refraction Over Current Lenses* on page 71.) If this results in excellent vision, only a change in the sphere needs be made.

As a general rule, **leaving the astigmatic part of a prescription unchanged** lessens the chance that there will be difficulty adjusting to the new prescription.

The corollary is also true: Changing the cylinder axis or power—especially the **axis**—increases the chance the patient will have difficulty adjusting to the new prescription.

Note

Another advantage of over-refraction is that the **vertex distance** (the distance between the glasses lens and cornea) is unlikely to be a factor with the new prescription. The new glasses will most likely sit in the same plane as the present glasses. The stronger the prescription, the more relevant vertex distance becomes.

Refraction Case 4

An 83-year-old male presents with 20/100 vision in each eye secondary to age-related macular degeneration. **Should the normal subjective refraction technique be modified when testing this patient?**

· · · · · ·
Answer

Yes. **Large changes** should be used when giving choices to a patient with low vision. When measuring power (both sphere and cylindrical), comparisons with a difference of 0.50 or 1.00 diopter can be shown. Axis choices can be followed by shifts of 15 degrees or greater.

Refraction Case 5

Two 70-year-old women present with the following best corrected visual acuity:

▶ **Patient 1: Distance vision of 20/30 with near vision of J1+ in each eye.**

▶ **Patient 2: Distance vision of 20/30 with near vision of J2 in each eye.**

Which patient is more likely to have age-related macular degeneration, and which is more likely to have a cataract?

· · · · · ·
Answer

Patient 1 is more likely to have a **cataract**. With an early to moderate cataract, there is often a disparity between distance and near acuity, with near better than distance.

Patient 2 is more likely to have **age-related macular degeneration**. With age-related macular degeneration, distance and near acuity tend to be comparable, most likely resulting from loss of foveal integrity.

Note
If a patient with decreased vision has both cataract and macular degeneration, this distinction can be helpful in determining which is more responsible for the decrease.

Refraction Case 6

A 78-year-old male is bothered by scratches on his lenses, and your refraction reveals that the measurements are unchanged. **You write a prescription that is identical to the previous one, but the patient finds that he cannot tolerate the new glasses.** When he returns, you put each pair of glasses in the lensometer and find that the measurement is the same. What should you do?

• • • • • •
Answer

The most likely explanation for his problem is that the **base curve** of the new lenses is different than that of the old pair. Often, the best way to resolve this is to have the patient take the old glasses to the optician along with your written request for the optician to "**duplicate the previous prescription, including duplication of the base curve.**"

Note

Similarly, if you would like to duplicate a patient's existing prism but are not completely sure you have measured it correctly in the present glasses, you can ask the optician to "**duplicate the prism.**"

Refraction Case 7

A 27-year-old female who does not wear glasses is having difficulty reading. What are the considerations?

. . . . . .
Answer

Reading difficulty in a 27-year-old patient is not due to presbyopia. Three primary considerations are as follows:

1. She may have **latent hyperopia**. If so, her accommodative ability is being used to correct the hyperopic refractive error, leaving an insufficient amount for reading.

2. **Convergence insufficiency**: The near point of convergence should be no farther away than 8 cm. Patients with convergence insufficiency typically complain of **headache** and **eye strain (asthenopia)**, which occur very soon after reading begins. Often, **words will begin to swim together**, and the patient should be asked whether this has been observed because it is quite diagnostic. **Convergence exercises** are a very effective treatment for these patients, with great success in eliminating their symptoms.

3. **Medication**: Medicines used for colds, motion sickness, and some central nervous system diseases are among those that can make reading more difficult by their effect on the pupil and accommodation. History is important in identifying this etiology.

Refraction Case 8

A 39-year-old female who has a -3.00 spherical myopic correction in each eye inquires about refractive surgery. When discussing the risks, benefits, and alternatives to surgery, what factors related to near vision should not be overlooked?

. . . . . .
Answer

Presbyopia should be explained to, and discussed with, the patient. She should understand that she will need to use reading glasses **in several years** if refractive surgery completely eliminates the nearsightedness in each eye. Reading glasses may not be necessary if the surgery is planned to provide monovision. (See *Refraction Case 9* on page 108.)

If the patient forgoes the surgery, she would retain the ability to read and see things at near with both eyes while not wearing glasses. Some presbyopic individuals find that ability valuable when doing various near tasks.

Refraction Case 9

A 55-year-old myopic male, who is a bifocal wearer, inquires about refractive surgery. What should you discuss?

. . . . . .
Answer

Remind the patient that there are essentially **"two prescriptions" in the bifocal glasses** he is now wearing: one for **distance** and the other for **near**. Discuss with him that if the distance vision is fully corrected in each eye, he will still need **glasses for reading**.

An alternative would be to have **monovision** laser correction, fully correcting one eye for distance while leaving the second eye with enough nearsightedness for reading and near activities. It should be pointed out to him that, with monovision, he will not be binocular, as one eye is blurred for distance and the other eye is blurred for near. A trial of monovison in contact lenses is very helpful prior to a decision about surgery.

The same considerations apply if he were a **PAL** wearer.

Refraction Case 10

An 80-year-old male comes into the examination room carrying a brown paper bag. He hands it to you saying, "Here are my glasses." Inside the bag, you find **seven pairs of glasses**. What do you do?

. . . . . .
Answer

The goal is to **simplify** things for the patient, and this will simplify things for you, too! It is helpful to ask:

▶ Is there one pair that you prefer?

▶ When do you use the other glasses? How old are the various pairs?

If he is using several pairs of glasses, each matched to a different activity, it may be appropriate to continue that way, but it is worthwhile to try to decrease the number. **The goal is to find the simplest system that satisfies the patient's visual needs.**

If most of the glasses are older prescriptions and are not being used, he should be encouraged to donate them to **The Lions Club** or other resource for distribution to the needy.

Refraction Case 11

A 75-year-old male who has needed OTC reading glasses for many years is surprised to find that he can now read without them. **Why are reading glasses no longer needed, and what is this phenomenon called?**

. . . . . .
Answer

The improvement in this patient's ability to read up close is not the result of regained accommodative ability. It is due to an increase in myopia, referred to as a **myopic shift**. It is this newly acquired nearsightedness that is allowing him to read unaided. The most common cause of a myopic shift is a **developing nuclear sclerotic cataract**. Another etiology is an **elevated blood glucose level** in an individual with diabetes mellitus.

Note

As a patient's near vision improves secondary to a myopic shift, there is a corresponding greater difficulty with distance vision due to the increased myopia.

Classically, when due to a cataract, this phenomenon has been called **second sight**.

Refraction Case 12

When fitting a contact lenses patient for monovision, it is necessary to know which eye is a patient's **dominant eye. How can this be determined?**

. . . . . .
Answer

There are a number of techniques for determining which eye is dominant. One easy method is to have the patient fully extend both arms with fingers overlapping and pointing upward. Above the overlapping thumbs, there should be a small opening.

Keeping both eyes open and with the arms outstretched, the patient is instructed to look at an object across the room through the small opening.

The examiner occludes one of the patient's eyes, and then the other. One eye will be able to see the object, and the other will not. **The eye that sees the object is the dominant eye.**

Note

The **dominant** eye will typically be fit with the contact lens for **distance**.

Refraction Case 13

A 13-year-old male is examined and found to be emmetropic. **At what age should he next be examined?**

• • • • • •
Answer

It is during the teenage years that myopia is most likely to develop. Because the change occurs gradually, teenagers may not be aware that they are seeing less well at distance. An examination every 1 or 2 years during this period is recommended.

Refraction Case 14

A 50-year-old female complains of **double vision**. When testing her acuity, it becomes apparent that she has **monocular diplopia** in the left eye. Could refractive error be the etiology of the double vision?

• • • • • •
Answer

Yes. **Uncorrected refractive error** usually results in a complaint of blurred vision, but can present as monocular diplopia. This symptom can occur when the sphere, cylinder, or axis is incorrect. It can also result from ocular surface abnormality, irregular astigmatism, or cataract (typically seen as ghosting). When a patient presents with monocular diplopia, a refraction should be performed. If the refractive result eliminates the double vision, the etiology has been determined.

Note

If the **pinhole test** eliminates the monocular diplopia, the most likely cause is refractive error, cataract, or ocular surface abnormality.

Special Considerations When Prescribing Glasses

Special Considerations Case 1

A 55-year-old male myope is examined and found to have a small change in his bifocal glasses prescription. He is planning to have it filled, but has **many questions**. How would you answer each?

1. Should my sunglasses also be updated?

2. If I get new sunglasses, I am going to get them without a bifocal. Can I use the same prescription?

3. What color should my sunglasses be?

4. Should I get the type of glasses that darken when I go outside?

5. Should I get an anti-glare coating on the new glasses?

6. Should my spare pair of glasses be updated?

7. I am going to be fit for contact lenses soon. Do I even need glasses?

8. Can I use the glasses prescription to get contact lenses?

9. Will you write me a prescription for contact lenses?

· · · · · ·
Answer

1. Should my **sunglasses** also be updated?

    With any change of glasses prescription, it is good to advise the patient to **have only one pair of glasses made initially**. Once the new pair of glasses is worn and found to be working well, additional pairs can be made.

    The patient can himself determine whether the sunglasses should be updated. He can do this by waiting until he receives his new glasses. Then, if he feels his vision with the existing sunglasses still seems satisfactory when **compared to his new glasses**, it is not essential that the sunglasses be changed. If he finds, by comparison, that he is no longer satisfied with the prescription in the sunglasses, they can be updated.

2. If I get new sunglasses, I am going to get them without a **bifocal**. Can I use the same prescription?

   A cautionary "Yes." The same prescription can be used, but **it is usually a good idea to get a bifocal or PAL in the sunglasses**. Although many activities outdoors do not require reading, it is beneficial to have the Add in sunglasses for looking at a map or cell phone when traveling, for reading at the beach, or for other outdoor situations requiring near viewing.

3. What **color** should my sunglasses be?

   Gray, as it is best for preserving natural colors.

4. Should I get the type of **glasses that darken when I go outside**?

   In the past, the reservations with photosensitive lenses were that they turned neither light enough indoors nor dark enough in the sun. Improvement in the lenses has greatly lessened these concerns. However, some patients still complain that the glasses do not get dark enough when **driving**. This is because the windshield absorbs a large percentage of the ultraviolet rays needed to cause the photochemical change.

5. Should I get an **anti-glare coating** on the new regular glasses?

   Many patients find two advantages of anti-glare coating:

   • The patient's own eyes are able to be seen clearly when the patient is speaking with another person, without **reflections** off the lenses obscuring them.

   • With **flash photography**, eyes are usually obscured by lens reflections in the absence of anti-glare coating.

6. Should my **spare pair of glasses** be updated?

   Initially, only one pair of glasses should be made. The patient should then test how he is seeing with the spare pair compared to the new glasses. If he feels he will still be able to **function satisfactorily with the spare pair** (despite the acuity not being as sharp as with the new prescription), then it is not necessary to update them. Using the older pair will not be causing any harm to his eyes.

Note

It may be helpful to the patient to suggest that he **keep the spare pair of glasses in his travel kit**. By doing so, he does not have to remember to pack them for traveling, and he will know where the glasses are should they be needed when at home.

7. I am going to be fit for **contact lenses** soon. Do I even need glasses?

   It is essential that all contact lens wearers have back-up glasses. Contact lenses are reasonably safe in eyes that are healthy. However, if a contact lens wearer develops conjunctivitis, a sty, or any other infection, the contact lenses must be discontinued. If there are no back-up glasses, some individuals will, with potentially serious consequences, continue wearing the contact lenses.

Alert

Infection and contact lenses do not mix; it is the ophthalmologic equivalent of drinking and driving.

8. Can I use the glasses prescription to get contact lenses?

   No, a glasses prescription is only a starting point for a contact lens fitting and cannot be used in lieu of it.

9. Will you write me a prescription for contact lenses?

   A proper contact lens prescription can be written **only after a contact lens fitting**.

Special Considerations Case 2

A 27-year-old male patient has **no light perception (NLP) in one eye due to an old injury and is emmetropic in the remaining eye**. What are your recommendations?

. . . .
Answer

Because he is functioning monocularly, it is important to maximally **protect the useful eye**. The patient should be encouraged to wear clear (plano) glasses with **poly-carbonate** or **Trivex lenses**. When playing a contact or racquet sport, **sports goggles** must be worn. Also, it should be recommended that the patient have a **yearly eye examination**. (See *Special Situations* on page 70.)

Special Considerations Case 3

A 57-year-old female is **NLP in one eye**, and refraction of her other eye results in a measurement of -3.25 -0.50 × 90° with a +2.50 Add. How should you write the prescription?

. . . .
Answer

For cosmetic purposes, it is desirable that the lens in front of the nonseeing eye be **similar in appearance** to the lens prescribed for the seeing eye. This is accomplished by writing the word "**balance**" on the prescription in the block where the spherical designation would normally be written. The optician will use a **balance lens** for the blind eye that will match the prescribed lens in thickness and style.

To protect the patient's only useful eye, **polycarbonate** or **Trivex lenses** should be specified on the glasses prescription, and she must wear **sports goggles** when playing any contact or racquet sport. Also, **yearly eye examinations** are recommended. (See *Special Situations* on page 70.)

Special Considerations Case 4

A 19-year-old female who has never worn glasses complains of a little difficulty seeing at distance. Refraction reveals a myopic correction in the **right eye** of **-1.50** and in the **left eye** of **-7.50**. **What is this called? What should you prescribe?**

• • • • • •
Answer

A significant difference in refractive error between the two eyes is called **anisometropia**.

If the refractive error in each eye were to be fully corrected, it would result in **aniseikonia**, a difference in image size. The more highly myopic eye (the left) would have a smaller image.

Usually, a difference in refractive error between the two eyes of **greater than 3.00 diopters** is not able to be fused, although the exact amount varies depending on the individual. A **trial run** can be very helpful in determining whether a significantly asymmetric prescription will be tolerated. (See *Trial Run* on page 68.) There are three ways to handle her anisometropia:

1. The left eye may be less than fully corrected, thus continuing to function as a "**spare tire**."

2. A **contact lens**, if used for the left eye, will eliminate the aniseikonia. It will do so because of the elimination of vertex distance as a factor.

3. Once the myopia is stable, **refractive surgery** could be considered.

Note

Anisometropic amblyopia is another consideration in this patient.

Special Considerations Case 5

An 80-year-old male with 20/40 vision in each eye secondary to **dry age-related macular degeneration** complains of **difficulty reading with his bifocal, which has a +2.50 Add**. What might you consider?

• • • • • •
Answer

An Add of +2.50 (or +3.00) is typically the maximum strength prescribed for a patient with normal visual acuity. However, a stronger Add than the norm can function as a low-vision aid.

This patient can be given a **+3.50** or **+4.00 Add** if he does not mind holding the reading material somewhat closer than he normally would. The increase in plus power results in a closer and narrower reading range.

If an **Add higher than +4.00** is decided upon, it is often best to give a separate pair of **single-vision reading glasses**. Again, the reading material would need to be held quite close.

> ### Note
> **Initially**, and especially if these measures do not work satisfactorily, consider referring him for consultation with a **Low Vision Service**.

Special Considerations Case 6

A 25-year-old female, who has not previously worn glasses, is refracted. She is found to have 20/20 vision in each eye with a measurement of **OD -2.50** and **OS plano**. What will you prescribe?

• • • • • •
Answer

This decision will depend on the **patient's preference**.

Without glasses, when viewing binocularly, she will see clearly at distance because the left eye is emmetropic. Thus, some individuals find that correcting the second eye does not add to their clarity, and they are happy to continue without glasses. Others, however, find that correction of the refractive error in the second eye gives a subjective improvement in acuity and prefer to have that eye corrected.

Note

The 2.50 diopter difference between the eyes **would not be expected to result in aniseikonia** and, therefore, glasses can be prescribed for this asymmetric prescription—after a trial run.

Special Considerations Case 7

A **55-year-old male's** refractive error is **OD -2.50** and **OS plano**. At present, he is **not wearing glasses. What will you prescribe?**

Answer

Unless he prefers to have each eye fully corrected at distance and near, he will continue to do well without glasses. He has "**natural monovision**," using the right eye for near and the left eye for distance.

If he would prefer to have the right eye corrected for distance, a bifocal or PAL will be needed because he is in the presbyopic age range.

If he is functioning well without glasses, it is best to do nothing.

Special Considerations Case 8

A 41-year-old female has only one pair of glasses. Refraction determines that she needs a change in each lens and you give her a prescription. She states that she **wants to use the same frames she now has,** but she cannot function without glasses and therefore cannot leave them with the optician. What might you recommend?

Answer

If the prescription is taken to an optical shop that will not have the new lenses available for several days, she can continue to wear her present glasses once the optician has determined the size of the lenses to be ordered. After the lab delivers the lenses to the optician, she can then return and have the old lenses removed and the new lenses inserted. (She should also keep the old lenses; it is always possible a new prescription will not be tolerated.)

Alternatively, if the prescription is taken to an optical shop that can make the new lenses while she waits, that would be a satisfactory solution.

Thus, there should not be a time when she would have to be without glasses.

Special Considerations Case 9

A 75-year-old male can no longer satisfactorily perform his activities of daily living secondary to **bilateral cataracts**. His best corrected visual acuities are OD 20/40 and OS 20/50. His cataracts have not caused a myopic shift, and his longstanding refractive correction is OD -3.50 and OS -3.50 +1.50 × 180°, with a +2.50 Add bilaterally.

He would like to have **cataract surgery** for the **left eye initially**, with subsequent surgery for his right eye. What are some **things to consider** with regard to postoperative refractive status?

• • • • • •
Answer

Some considerations are as follows:

If he chooses to have a **monofocal intraocular lens implant** for his left eye, he will need to decide if he wants that eye to see well unaided, at **distance**, **near**, or **in-between**.

A **toric intraocular lens** (if the astigmatism is corneal rather than lenticular) can be considered for the left eye.

Another alternative is to plan for **monovision**—one eye for distance, the other for near. Prior to making a decision about this option, it is good to do a monovision trial with a contact lens.

If he would prefer to have a **multifocal** or **accommodating** intraocular lens implant for his left eye, he will not have to choose between distance and near vision. However, he should be made aware of the possibility of glare, decrease in contrast sensitivity, and visual acuity compromise with the current generation of multifocal lenses. When considering an accommodating lens, the amount of accommodation achievable should be discussed.

If he chooses to have an implant that will eliminate the myopia in his left eye, **aniso-metropia** will be a consideration for the **interval between** the first and second surgeries. (See *Special Considerations Case 4* on page 115.) If he were to have difficulty during this period due to the asymmetric refractive error, a **contact lens** could be used in the right eye to eliminate the disparity in image size.

Special Considerations Case 10

A 65-year-old male, who was seen 1 year prior, is complaining of blurred vision. He is refracted and found to have had a **change in spherical power**, **cylinder axis**, and **cylinder power** in each eye. His right eye has an upper lid **chalazion**, and the left eye has upper lid **ptosis**. Could either of these be responsible for the change in refractive error?

• • • • • •
Answer

Yes, each can be responsible for the measured change.

Both a **chalazion** and a **ptotic upper lid** can push on the cornea and produce **irregular astigmatism** (principal meridians not 90 degrees apart). Best corrected visual acuity may be decreased, but it will improve on pinhole testing. After corrective surgery is performed, the cornea is expected to return, slowly, to its prior shape.

Special Considerations Case 11

A 65-year-old female's visual acuity is measured while she is wearing her **PAL glasses**, and she is found to have decreased vision at distance in each eye. Her subsequent eye examination reveals no abnormal findings. What are two **glasses-related causes** that are not infrequently encountered?

• • • • • •
Answer

One possible cause is simply that her **lenses are not clean**. Another is that she may be looking at distance through the **lower portion** (the progression) of the PAL glasses, either because her **chin is elevated** or because the **occluder has pushed the glasses upward** on her face. It is easy to rectify these causes and then retest acuity.

Appendix

Kolker RJ, Kolker AF. *Subjective Refraction and
Prescribing Glasses: The Number One (or Number Two)
Guide to Practical Techniques and Principles (pp 121-129).*
© 2018 Taylor & Francis Group.

HOW TO USE THE MANUAL LENSOMETER

Plus Cylinder Method

Prior to Measuring

1. Make sure the prism knob is straight up (at 90) and positioned at zero. (For a progressive addition lens [PAL], which should be measured at the top of the lens, the prism knob can be used to accomplish the centering.)

2. Before the glasses are placed in the lensometer, look through the ocular and turn it so the numbers/circles are in focus.

3. Place the glasses, with the arms pointing away, flat on the adjustable shelf. (The axis measurement will be incorrect if the glasses are not level.)

4. The intersection of the lines (the optical center of the lens) should be positioned within the central circle.

5. Naming the lines can be a source of confusion. We will call the three thin lines that are very close together "the single line." We will call the three thicker lines spaced farther apart "the three lines."

Steps for Measuring the Prescription

1. Begin to straighten and focus the single line but, while doing so, check ("peek") to make sure the three lines are going to be in focus in the plus direction, with the dial turning counterclockwise. If the three lines are coming into focus moving in the clockwise direction, change the axis of the single line by 90 degrees.

2. Focus and align the single line; this measures the spherical power and the cylinder axis, respectively.

3. Focus the three lines by turning the knob counterclockwise. When the three lines are in focus, determine the dioptric difference between the measurement of the single line and the three lines; this is the amount of plus cylinder power.

When an Add is present, there is a fourth step:

4. Elevate the shelf and focus/straighten the single line in the Add segment. The dioptric difference between the measurement of the single line in the distance portion of the lens and in the Add segment is the amount of the Add.

Note

In a PAL, there is almost always a laser marking indicating the strength of the Add located at the lower outer portion of the lens, often below a manufacturer's insignia. This can be read with the help of background illumination provided by an overhead room light.

When measuring a high plus or high minus lens, a different technique is used when measuring the Add. The glasses are repositioned in the lensometer with the arms pointing toward you. The single line is measured both in the distance and near sections, with the difference being the strength of the Add.

When learning to read prism in glasses, practice with known prisms from the trial lens set.

HOW TO USE THE MANUAL LENSOMETER

Minus Cylinder Method

Prior to Measuring

1. Make sure the prism knob is straight up (at 90) and positioned at zero. (For a PAL, which should be measured at the top of the lens, the prism knob can be used to accomplish the centering.)

2. Before the glasses are placed in the lensometer, look through the ocular and turn it so the numbers/circles are in focus.

3. Place the glasses, with the arms pointing away, flat on the adjustable shelf. (The axis measurement will be incorrect if the glasses are not level.)

4. The intersection of the lines (the optical center of the lens) should be positioned within the central circle.

5. Naming the lines can be as source of confusion. We will call the three thin lines that are very close together "the single line." We will call the three thicker lines spaced farther apart "the three lines."

Steps for Measuring the Prescription

1. Begin to straighten and focus the single line but, while doing so, check ("peek") to make sure the three lines are going to be in focus in the minus direction, with the dial turning clockwise. If the three lines are coming into focus moving in the counterclockwise direction, change the axis of the single line by 90 degrees.

2. Focus and align the single line; this measures the spherical power and the cylinder axis, respectively.

3. Focus the three lines by turning the knob clockwise. When the three lines are in focus, determine the dioptric difference between the measurement of the single line and the three lines; this is the amount of minus cylinder power.

When an Add is present, there is a fourth step:

4. Elevate the shelf and focus/straighten the single line in the Add segment. The dioptric difference between the measurement of the single line in the distance portion of the lens and in the Add segment is the amount of the Add.

Note

In a PAL, there is almost always a laser marking indicating the strength of the Add located at the lower outer portion of the lens, often below a manufacturer's insignia. This can be read with the help of background illumination provided by an overhead room light.

When measuring a high plus or high minus lens, a different technique is used when measuring the Add. The glasses are repositioned in the lensometer with the arms pointing toward you. The single line is measured both in the distance and near sections, with the difference being the strength of the Add.

When learning to read prism in glasses, practice with known prisms from the trial lens set.

RETINOSCOPY PRIMER

Plus Cylinder Method

Preparation

▶ Room lights are dim, not off.

▶ Use a projected dot as the distance fixation target (accommodation less likely).

▶ The working distance = arm's length from patient (66 cm).

The Retinoscope

▶ Right hand for right eye, left hand for left eye.

▶ Your right eye is aligned with the patient's right eye, and vice versa for left.

▶ Use the widest streak/beam, thumb slide up or down depending on model.

▶ Two maneuvers:

  • Turning sleeve to view reflexes at perpendicular axes

  • Sweeping side to side (with streak vertical) and up and down (with streak horizontal) to observe movement of reflex

▶ Note: If there is an oblique cylinder, you can sweep in diagonal positions (90 degrees apart).

▶ Movement of reflex (streak) seen within pupil when sweeping can be as follows:

  • With = Reflex moves in the same direction as sweep

  • Against = Reflex moves in the opposite direction of sweep

  • No movement (the reflex fills the pupil) = Neutralization

Procedure

▶ The goal of retinoscopy is neutralization of the two reflexes—they are 90 degrees apart.

▶ The sequence is identical to that of subjective refraction: sphere, cylinder axis, cylinder power, sphere!

After obtaining the red reflex:

1. Move the sphere dial in the minus direction until you see "with" movement at 90 and 180 degrees.

2. Sweep, alternating at 90 and 180 degrees, while adding plus sphere power until the first axis is neutralized. (The remaining un-neutralized axis will still be in the plus direction and will have "with" movement) = Working sphere power

3. Turn the axis knob on the phoropter to the position of the remaining un-neutralized axis. (It will be perpendicular to the location of the neutralized axis) = Cylinder axis

4. Add plus cylinder power until the "with" reflex at the cylinder axis is neutralized = Cylinder power

5. Subtract 1.50 diopters (for the working distance) from the sphere found in Step 2 = Final sphere power

Note

Retinoscopy after cycloplegia is a good way to begin learning.

For children who cannot sit behind a phoropter, hand-held trial lenses can be used.

When neutralizing "with" reflexes, move in larger diopter steps initially, then smaller ones.

Oblique cylinder will tilt the reflex away from 90 and 180 degrees. Narrowing the streak briefly can help localize an oblique axis. Work with axes 90 degrees apart.

Record your retinoscopy findings for comparison with the final subjective refraction.

Practice.

RETINOSCOPY PRIMER

Minus Cylinder Method

Preparation

► Room lights are dim, not off.

► Use a projected dot as the distance fixation target (accommodation less likely).

► The working distance = arm's length from patient (66 cm).

The Retinoscope

► Right hand for right eye, left hand for left eye.

► Your right eye is aligned with the patient's right eye, and vice versa for left.

► Use the widest streak/beam, thumb slide up or down depending on model.

► Two maneuvers:

• Turning sleeve to view reflexes at perpendicular axes

• Sweeping side to side (with streak vertical) and up and down (with streak horizontal) to observe movement of reflex

► Note: If there is an oblique cylinder, you can sweep in diagonal positions (90 degrees apart).

► Movement of reflex (streak) seen within pupil when sweeping can be as follows:

• With = Reflex moves in the same direction as sweep

• Against = Reflex moves in the opposite direction of sweep

• No movement (the reflex fills the pupil) = Neutralization

Procedure

▸ The goal of retinoscopy is neutralization of the two reflexes—they are 90 degrees apart.

▸ The sequence is identical to that of subjective refraction: sphere, cylinder axis, cylinder power, sphere!

After obtaining the red reflex:

1. Move the sphere dial in the minus direction until you see "with" movement at 90 and 180 degrees.

2. Sweep, alternating at 90 and 180 degrees, while adding plus sphere power until the second axis is neutralized. (The first axis to neutralize will now be in the minus direction and will have "against" movement) = Working sphere power

3. Turn the axis knob on the phoropter to the position where the first axis was neutralized. (It will be perpendicular to the location of the neutralized second axis) = Cylinder axis

4. Add minus cylinder power until the "against" reflex at the cylinder axis is neutralized = Cylinder power

5. Subtract 1.50 diopters (for the working distance) from the sphere found in Step 2 = Final sphere power

Note

Retinoscopy after cycloplegia is a good way to begin learning.

For children who cannot sit behind a phoropter, hand-held trial lenses can be used.

When neutralizing "with" and "against" reflexes, move in larger diopter steps initially, then smaller ones.

Oblique cylinder will tilt the reflex away from 90 and 180 degrees. Narrowing the streak briefly can help localize an oblique axis. Work with axes 90 degrees apart.

Record your retinoscopy findings for comparison with the final subjective refraction.

Practice.

Index